EMERGENCY MEDICINE PEARLS

EMERGENCY MEDICINE PEARLS

Second Edition

ADAM J. SINGER, MD

Associate Professor
Department of Emergency Medicine
State University of New York
Stony Brook, New York

JONATHAN L. BURSTEIN, MD

Assistant Professor of Medicine
Harvard Medical School
Harvard University
Boston, Massachusetts

FREDERICK M. SCHIAVONE, MD

Residency Director
Associate Professor
Department of Emergency Medicine
State University of New York
Stony Brook, New York

F.A. DAVIS COMPANY • Philadelphia

F.A. Davis Company
1915 Arch Street
Philadelphia, PA 19103

Printed in Canada

Last digit indicates print number: 10 9 8 7 6 5 4 3

Senior Medical Editor: Robert W. Reinhardt
Senior Developmental Editor: Bernice M. Wissler
Production Editor: Stephen Johnson
Cover Designer: Louis J. Forgione

Library of Congress Cataloging-in-Publication Data

Singer, Adam J.
    Emergency medicine pearls / Adam J. Singer, Jonathan
L. Burstein, Frederick M. Schiavone.— 2nd ed.
        p. ; cm.
    Includes index.
    ISBN 0-8036-0755-5
    1. Emergency medicine—Handbooks, manuals, etc.
2. Residents (Medicine)—Handbooks, manuals, etc.
I. Burstein, Jonathan L. II. Schiavone, Frederick M. III. Title.
    [DNLM: 1. Emergency Medicine—methods—Handbooks.
2. Emergencies—Handbooks. WB 39 S617e 2000]
RC86.8 .S58 2000
616.02′5—dc21

                                    00-059039

As new scientific information becomes available through basic and clinical research, recommended treatments and drug therapies undergo changes. The authors and publisher have done everything possible to make this book accurate, up to date, and in accord with accepted standards at the time of publication. The authors, editors, and publisher are not responsible for errors or omissions or for consequences from application of the book, and make no warranty, expressed or implied, in regard to the contents of the book. Any practice described in this book should be applied by the reader in accordance with professional standards of care used in regard to the unique circumstances that may apply in each situation. The reader is advised always to check product information (package inserts) for changes and new information regarding dose and contraindications before administering any drug. Caution is especially urged when using new or infrequently ordered drugs.

Preface to the Second Edition

We are pleased to present the second edition of *Emergency Medicine Pearls*. In this edition, several notable changes have been made. First, we have added "Prehospital Considerations," a section for prehospital providers, who, along with medical students and residents, have found our book useful. Second, we have incorporated specific pearls within the text in boldface type to facilitate their use. Third, we have significantly updated many of the chapters and have included new diagnostic approaches, such as spiral CT angiography for pulmonary embolism, as well as new therapies, such as thrombolytics for ischemic stroke, glycoprotein IIb/IIIa inhibitors for acute coronary syndromes, and new antibiotic regimens for infectious diseases. Finally, a new chapter about common ear, nose, and throat problems, such as earache and epistaxis, has been incorporated into this edition of *Emergency Medicine Pearls*. We hope that our readers will find these changes helpful.

Preface to the First Edition

Emergency medicine became a specialty in the early 1970s. Since then, many fine textbooks on emergency medicine have been published. However, much of the information available is not always practical and applicable to specific clinical conditions. Also, it is impossible to read and digest all of this information in a timely manner before one begins working in the emergency department. These texts, while preparing emergency medicine residents for specialty boards, do not help them prepare for the first few months in the emergency department.

We wrote this manual for the junior emergency medicine resident as well as for rotating medical students, interns, and residents in other departments. Using a practical, simple approach, we cover the majority of acute problems encountered in a busy emergency department. We also cover several issues not always well addressed in other texts, such as how to prepare for an incoming patient with a cardiac arrest, what information to obtain from prehospital personnel, what "labs" to order and when, and how to tell a family that their loved one has died.

Emergency Medicine Pearls is very easy to read and may be completed in a few hours, such as on the night before your "tour of duty" in the emergency department. Although some of our recommendations are controversial, we usually have chosen to address commonly encountered problems so that the inexperienced practitioner will at least have some idea of what to do, especially under the sometimes stressful conditions in the emergency department.

We did not intend for this manual to replace information included in more comprehensive textbooks; it may not improve your grades on the in-service exam or the specialty boards. Instead, we offer general guidelines and clinical pearls to help you deal with some of the more common problems early in your career, and thus minimize your already stressful beginning.

Adam J. Singer, MD
Jonathan L. Burstein, MD
Frederick M. Schiavone, MD

Contents

1
CHAPTER

Welcome to the Emergency Department

The white rabbit put on his spectacles. "Where shall I begin, please your majesty?" he asked. "Begin at the beginning," the King said gravely, "and go on till you come to the end; then stop."

Lewis Carroll

The emergency department (ED) is a chaotic place. You may feel that you're in Wonderland, and that everyone around you is as mad as a hatter . . . but if you pay attention, patterns will emerge. We hope that this book will reveal some of these patterns before you start, making your beginning in emergency medicine easier.

The ED and its staff are dedicated to the patients streaming through every day: the sick, the injured, and those with nowhere else to turn. When they enter the ED, they are first evaluated by the triage nurse. Based on the patients' chief complaints and vital signs, they are then divided into those requiring immediate care, those requiring urgent care, and those who can safely wait. The triage nurse will notify the physician-in-charge of any patient requiring immediate attention. Everyone else gets seen in order of urgency and presentation. Usually, there is a chart rack or box into which the paperwork is placed to indicate that a patient is ready to be seen by a physician. Your job will most likely be to pick up the next chart in the rack and see that patient.

INITIAL ASSESSMENT

For all of these patients, the emergency physician must answer two questions: (1) Does this patient have a life-threatening condition? and (2) Where should this patient go? Keep these questions in mind when you see a patient; the person doing triage is not perfect, and patients' conditions may change while they are waiting to be seen. Before you go through the detailed history and physical (H&P), which is the usual routine of other specialties, ask yourself if there is something you must do now to resuscitate and stabilize the patient. Sometimes this is obvious: the teenager with a sprained ankle (you have time); the elderly man in cardiac arrest (you must act). Sometimes it's trickier: the 70-year-old woman who comes in confused; the motorcyclist thrown 20 feet through the air who is complaining of abdominal pain. When in doubt, ask the supervising physician to sort out who needs immediate intervention. Always look at the patient's vital signs (usually obtained by the triage nurse; if not, get them yourself). Make sure that all four vital signs are measured (heartbeat, body temperature, respiration, and blood pressure). Marked abnormalities must be explained and addressed in some way. Also, look carefully at the patient as you enter the room; with experience, this initial impression can tell you most of what you need to know.

FURTHER ASSESSMENT

Let us now assume that the patient is sufficiently stable for you to begin your detailed assessment. Keep in mind that you'll do a concise form of the H&P. The ED H&P is "directed" to the chief complaint and should be short and concise, but inclusive. Certain situations mandate specific detail. In patients with chest pain, a smoking history (as well as other cardiac risk factors) is relevant; in the woman with right upper quadrant abdominal pain, a history of recent gonorrhea may lead you down a particular path (specifically Fitz Hugh-Curtis syndrome). With experience and training, you will learn the relevant questions and physical findings. The streamlining of your H&P will serve you in other settings as well. Always note what the patient's chief complaint is. It will have to be addressed in your workup and write-up. **PEARL: It is very important to find out whether the "true" complaint differs from the written chief complaint.** For example, a patient may complain of headache, but his or her real question is, "Do I have a brain tumor?" If you do not ascertain this concern and deal with it, the patient will be upset and the workup and disposition will likely be hindered. Sometimes, the true complaint will come up while you are taking your history; at other times, you may need to elicit it with such questions as, "What concerns you the most?" or "How do you expect we'll be able to help you best?" Of course, be careful not to ask these in a challenging manner. Also, be sure to read nurses' notes or prehospital-care notes.

MANAGEMENT DECISIONS

Now that you have completed the H&P, you should have a pretty good idea of what is wrong with the patient. In most cases, your disposition will be decided based on the H&P. In the remaining cases, the next step is to decide what lab tests or consultations are needed to determine your differential diagnosis. Also, decide what procedures will be necessary to manage the patient's problem. Does a laceration need to be sutured? Do you need to see an electrocardiogram (ECG) to decide what to do next? In most EDs, at this point you will write orders for the interventions, medications, tests, or x-rays you want and then communicate with the nurses and ancillary staff to get these things done. Some things you will usually need to do yourself (e.g., suturing).

Note that the nursing staff and others are valuable assets for the patient's care. Each person usually has specific duties in the care of the patient, and you will find that they will be far more helpful to you if you work closely and cooperatively with them and include them in the treatment plan. If something must get done soon and you cannot do it yourself, talk with the nurse who is taking care of the patient about what needs to be done. (You may find that he or she is already doing it.) Pay attention to the nurse's assessment of the patient, usually documented in a nursing note; you will often find valuable information that you did not pick up before.

A few tips on labwork: If you do not know what to order, ask somebody, such as the attending physician. **PEARL: When in doubt, remember the "survival kit" of ECG, chest x-ray, and arterial blood gases (ABGs)—the information gained will usually rapidly reassure you or point you toward a diagnosis.** (Be careful not to indiscriminately "shotgun" labs, because this often complicates rather than simplifies the workup.) When drawing blood, draw one of each type of tube, if possible. It may save the patient a restick later if it turns out that other lab tests are necessary. Putting in a heparin lock and drawing the blood through it can save the patient from a second stick for intravenous (IV) access.

PEARL: Order labs early. Sometimes, the patient's disposition depends on lab results, which may take several hours to return; the sooner they are sent, the sooner you will be able to make an appropriate disposition for the patient. In many cases, other services will need to be involved; this is discussed later in this chapter.

Reaching an exact diagnosis in the ED is often not possible or expected. The definitive lab results or procedures, such as blood culture results or an exercise test, may not be available. Nevertheless, make an effort to assign a working diagnosis to your patient, both to guide your workup and to aid you in making the appropriate disposition or involving the right consultant. You will become skilled in making a diagnosis with very little information. Using pattern recognition is a valuable tool. For example, in an elderly person with carotid bruits (hence, atherosclerotic disease) and abdominal pain, the astute clinician will at least consider the presence of ischemic bowel.

MANAGEMENT AND DISPOSITION OF THE PATIENT

The next step is the disposition of the patient. You have only a few options: send the patient home, admit the patient to the hospital floors or intensive care unit (ICU), or observe the patient in the ED for a short time, most often not more than several hours. This decision can sometimes be made with only a few test results, although in many EDs the "admitting labs" will be sent off if a patient is clearly going to be admitted, as a courtesy to the admitting service.

Consulting Other Services

At this juncture, other services (e.g., cardiology or surgery) may be involved in the care of the patient, usually in one of three ways:

- The patient is going to be admitted to that service.
- The service will be asked to see the patient in follow-up after discharge.
- Specific procedures or advice will be obtained from the service to allow discharge of the patient (e.g., plastic surgery to repair a complex facial laceration).

Specific methods for contacting other services will vary from place to place, as will the political complications (no one likes being called by the ED—it means more work!). The ED attending physician is your best guide through these thickets. In general, when calling other services, be brief, make it clear why you are calling, and have all relevant data in front of you for rapid reference (e.g., H&P notes, labs, ECGs, or old chart). If a patient has a primary physician, it is appropriate (and almost mandatory), if possible, to let that person know what your plan is. The primary physician may be a useful source of information about the patient as well.

DOCUMENTATION

ED notes tend to be brief and full of abbreviations, but keep in mind that they are medicolegal documents, just as all medical records are. Always document your thought processes, include pertinent positive and negative findings in your note, and write short continuation notes documenting repeat examinations or responses to therapy. Remember the old adage, "not written means not done." You may be convinced that the 30-year-old man with pleuritic right-sided sharp chest pain has no cardiac problems, but picture the scene in court after he drops dead of a heart attack, and your note is found to read: "30 male chest pain. Lungs clear. Heart RRR no m/g/r." Why didn't you order an ECG? Why were you so convinced his pain was noncardiac? Your notes should reflect this. Being concise does not mean being incomplete. **PEARL: Warning: do not let**

your zeal for documentation disrupt patient care. In most cases, there is ample time to complete notes after the patient is stabilized and the disposition is established. With time and practice, you'll find that you can write better and better notes in less and less time.

DISCHARGING THE PATIENT

For patient discharge, four steps are necessary:

1. **Follow-up.** Arrange follow-up instructions for all discharged patients. This can be as simple as telling the patient to call his or her own doctor if any problems occur. In general, anyone sent home with a potentially serious problem, such as chest pain or abdominal pain, should be given very clear instructions regarding what specific problems need a doctor's attention, whom to see or call, and when to call. Whenever possible, contact the physician you want the patient to see in follow-up to ensure that these instructions can be carried out in a timely manner. **PEARL: You must provide an interpreter for non–English-speaking patients. If no one is available (e.g., a friend, relative, or staff member), a long-distance telephone carrier is usually able to provide this service.**

2. **Warning signs.** Remember that your diagnosis may be wrong or the patient's condition may deteriorate. Therefore, give all patients a list of problems or warning signs that require immediate return to the ED. For example, a patient with right lower quadrant pain, who seems well enough to go home but might conceivably have appendicitis, could be told: "If the pain becomes more severe or you develop repeated vomiting or fever, come back here immediately."

3. **Medication.** Specify what medication should be taken, and give specific instructions regarding how and when to take medications. **PEARL: Avoid the use of medical abbreviations. Don't write doses and timing of medications in medical "jargon."** Avoid terms such as bid, tid, and q/h.

4. **Specific instructions.** Give specific instructions regarding allowable or desirable activities and diet, as well as use of special measures (e.g., ice pack, heating pads), as appropriate.

Some EDs provide preprinted or computer-generated discharge instructions for particular problems; these should be used if available, because they undoubtedly will be more detailed than your own written instructions.

SIGNING OUT

At the beginning and end of each shift, you will go through a ritual handing-off of responsibility for patients, known as "sign-out." When you are leaving, it's a good idea to prepare for this. Check all of your patients' charts to ensure that you've written your note, make all the telephone calls or consult calls you can (because you know the patient best), and make sure that the workup (e.g., labs, x-rays) is being carried out. Before signing out, walk by the rooms to check that you haven't forgotten a particular patient (yes, this happens!). At sign-out, make sure the oncoming person who will take over for your patient knows what has been done, what needs to be done, and what you think is going on with the patient. Conversely, when you are coming in, make sure that you get all this information, and ask for it if you don't get it. Smooth sign-outs are vital for proper patient care and flow!

WHAT YOU WEAR AND CARRY

While you are working in the ED, what you wear and carry can make a difference in your ability to do your job. Clothing should be neat, clean, and functional. Avoid necklaces, dangling earrings, scarves, and ties (in most places); patients or visitors with behavioral problems may grab these, seriously injuring you in the process. Also avoid wearing anything of great value, such as an expensive watch or Grandma's ring. They could easily be damaged or stolen in the hectic environment of the ED. Always wear comfortable shoes—as an experiment, try wearing poorly fitting shoes for one shift and see how you feel!

Equipment you burden yourself with should serve a real purpose. In most cases, you won't need a tuning fork or ophthalmoscope; the first is seldom needed, and the second is usually mounted on the wall in each room. A good stethoscope is vital, and it is the only piece of equipment many ED physicians carry. It can also double as a reflex hammer. A good penlight can be useful—even more so a working pen (but a cheap one, because it may very well end up permanently "borrowed"). A good pair of heavy-duty shears is quite helpful ("paramedic shears") for cutting bandages, clothing, and so on. Using index cards to keep track of each patient will help you to keep your thoughts organized. Most important, bring your wits, enthusiasm, and energy—you will find them taxed but stimulated in the organized chaos of the ED.

2
CHAPTER

Know Your ABCs: Resuscitation and Stabilization

The ABCs in emergency medicine form the basic approach to all patients in the ED, no matter how trivial the presenting complaint seems. ABC stands for *airway, breathing,* and *circulation*. By performing a rapid ABC assessment for every patient, you minimize your chances of missing a life-threatening problem.

Although the ABCs are presented in a sequential manner in order of priorities, remember that emergency medicine is a team effort. Therefore, often all three aspects are addressed simultaneously.

PREHOSPITAL CONSIDERATIONS

▸ Most patients with severe alteration in their ABCs are brought to the ED by emergency medical service (EMS).
▸ EMS personnel must present all the necessary information about the patient's condition.
▸ Always use 100% oxygen in the resuscitation of these patients (there is no place for 2L nasal cannula).
▸ Rapid establishment of IV access and cardiac monitoring should be performed on all unstable patients.

AIRWAY

We cannot over-emphasize the importance of assessing and managing a patient's airway. **PEARL: Anticipate the need for active airway management, and reassess the airway continuously.** Assessment begins as the patient enters the room:

- Is the patient able to talk?
- Does the patient have hoarseness, stridor, or cyanosis?
- Does the patient have any suprasternal, intercostal, or subcostal retractions?
- Is the patient breathing?
- Are there obvious facial fractures, broken teeth, or particles of vomitus in the patient's mouth?

The most common cause of upper airway obstruction in the supine unconscious patient is posterior displacement of the base of the tongue, usually in the patient with an altered mental status. Therefore, start by opening the airway and bringing the tongue forward. This is best accomplished using a combined head tilt and chin lift (Fig. 2–1). When cervical spine (C-spine) injury is suspected, immobilize the neck (e.g., with a hard collar, head blocks) and perform a jaw thrust (Fig. 2–2). Avoid moving the neck. Open the mouth and look for any obvious causes of obstruction, such as broken teeth, dentures, foreign bodies, or vomitus. Use a hard-tipped suction catheter to clean out the mouth. If the patient starts breathing more easily, you may want to insert an oral or nasopharyngeal airway, as tolerated by the patient.

Intubation

Patients with a compromised airway need definitive airway management by endotracheal intubation or establishment of a surgical airway. *As a rule, anyone who can tolerate it should be intubated.* Indications for intubation include:

- Apnea
- Airway obstruction
- Respiratory failure
- Risk of aspiration in a patient with an altered mental state
- The need for hyperventilation in patients with severe

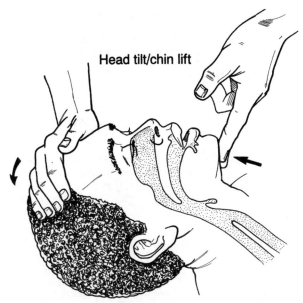

Head tilt/chin lift

Figure 2–1. The head-tilt/chin-lift maneuver. Tilt the head backward with one hand, while the other hand lifts the chin forward.

head injuries, usually with Glasgow Coma Scale (GCS) score < 8 (see Table 3–2)
• Combative patient (to avoid further injury)
The decision to intubate should be based on clinical grounds. **PEARL: Do not rely on arterial blood gas values (ABGs) or a chest x-ray to determine the patient's need for intubation. Use your clinical judgment.** The biggest pitfall in airway management is failing to intubate the patient in a timely fashion.

Anticipating a Difficult Intubation

The following clinical parameters suggest that intubation will be technically difficult:
• Short neck
• Buck teeth
• Large tongue

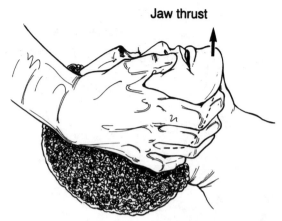

Figure 2–2. In the jaw-thrust maneuver, *place your fingers be-hind the angle of the patient's jaw and forcefully bring it forward.*

- Short distance between the tip of the chin and thyroid cartilage [<3 finger breadths (Fig. 2–3)]

If any of these is present, you may want to call for backup (e.g., an anesthesiologist) or prepare for a surgical airway by needle cricothyroidotomy or cricothyroidotomy. **PEARL: Always anticipate a difficult intubation, and be prepared to use an adjunct technique.**

Methods of Airway Management

Although most textbooks emphasize the technique of endotracheal intubation, *it is important to spend time mas-tering the proper use of the bag valve mask (BVM).* To be ef-fective, it is often necessary for two people to perform BVM ventilation. The BVM enables both oxygenation and ventilation of the patient when you are unable to intubate the patient immediately, and it allows time to mobilize personnel more experienced in airway management. Re-member that the airway remains unprotected from aspi-ration when a BVM is used, and *proper head positioning is required to minimize inadvertent ventilation of the stomach.* The major difficulty when using the BVM is maintaining a good mask seal; therefore, the two-handed method is most effective (Fig. 2–4).

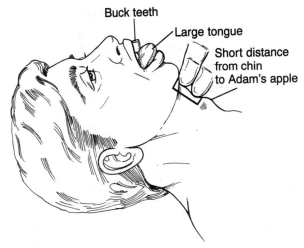

Buck teeth

Large tongue

Short distance from chin to Adam's apple

Figure 2–3. Anatomic features of a difficult airway.

Rapid-Sequence Induction Intubation

PEARL: The most useful tool for emergency endotracheal intubation is rapid-sequence induction (RSI). In RSI, general anesthesia and neuromuscular blockade are induced to achieve optimum intubating conditions and patient control while maintaining maximum protection against aspiration. Always assume that the patient has a full stomach. Also, be prepared to establish a surgical airway if intubation is unsuccessful. The patient should not be ventilated with a BVM before the initial attempt to intubate. This helps to prevent gastric distention and passive regurgitation during the procedure.

The sequence of RSI may be remembered using the "Five Ps":

1. **Preoxygenate:** If possible, give O_2 via a nonrebreather mask for 5 minutes. This builds an O_2 reserve that allows apnea for 3 to 5 minutes.
2. **Prepare the following:**
   a. Suction (hard-tipped Yankauer catheter in case of regurgitation).
   b. Two working IV lines.
   c. Monitors (cardiac, pulse oximeter, end-tidal CO_2).

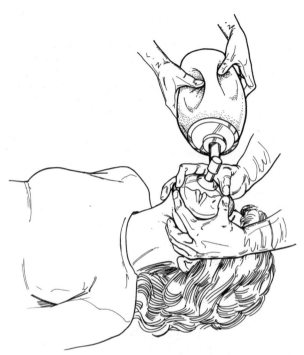

Figure 2–4. The two-handed technique: One rescuer achieves a tight two-handed seal with the mask, while the other rescuer squeezes the bag.

    d. Laryngoscope (fresh batteries and bulb).
    e. Blades—a #3 or #4 Macintosh for most adults, a #2 Miller for children < 8 years, or a #1 Miller for infants.
    f. Endotracheal tubes: men, 7.0 to 8.5 mm; women, 6.5 to 8.0 mm. In children > 1 year, the size of the endotracheal tube may be estimated by using the following formula:

$$\text{Tube size} = 4 + \frac{\text{Child's age}}{4}$$

    g. Stylet (this should not protrude through the end of the tube).
    h. BVM, connected to 100% O_2.

    i. Direct a nurse to draw up all drugs and label them appropriately.

    j. Have a cricothyroidotomy set available and opened.

    k. Patient positioning: align the oropharyngeal–laryngeal axis by placing the patient in the "sniffing" position (neck flexed, head extended). The patient's head should be raised 2 to 4 inches by placing a pad or a blanket under the head (Fig. 2–5). *Do not move the patient's head if cervical trauma is suspected.*

3. **Pretreat:** Lidocaine 1 mg/kg by IV push (IVP) may blunt the sudden rise in intracranial pressure (ICP) induced by laryngoscopy and intubation. You may use vecuronium 1 mg IVP (0.01 mg/kg) as a defasciculating dose before using a depolarizing paralytic agent to avoid fasciculations.

4. **Induce and paralyze:**

    a. Induce with etomidate 20 mg IVP (0.3 mg/kg), thiopental 350 to 500 mg IVP (3 to 5 mg/kg), or mi-

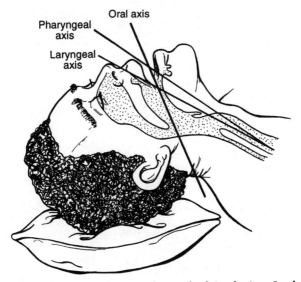

Figure 2–5. Head positioning for tracheal intubation. In the sniffing position, the neck is flexed while the head is extended. This creates the shortest distance and straightest line between the mouth and the vocal cords.

dazolam 5 mg IVP (0.1 to 0.2 mg/kg). You may omit induction if the patient is comatose.

b. Paralyze with either succinylcholine 120 mg IVP (1.5 mg/kg) or vecuronium 10 mg IVP (0.1 mg/kg). Children under 5 years old should receive atropine 0.02 mg/kg IV (minimum dose 0.1 mg) to avoid bradycardia. Rocuronium and mivacurium are newer nondepolarizing paralytic agents that are useful because of their rapid onset and reasonable duration.

c. Perform the Sellick maneuver. After giving the induction agent, have an assistant apply pressure with thumb and index finger to the cricoid cartilage. This compresses and occludes the esophagus against the C-spine to avoid passive gastroesophageal reflux and aspiration (Fig. 2–6). It may also push the cords down into view with a very anterior larynx. Apply cricoid pressure at the onset of apnea and maintain it until endotracheal tube placement is confirmed. If active esophageal regurgitation occurs, you must release cricoid pressure.

5. **Pass the tube:** Proceed with intubation after confirming that the following conditions exist: apnea, lack of eyelid twitch upon stimulation, and flaccidity of the jaw. Insert the blade of the laryngoscope into the right corner of the mouth and push the tongue to the left (Fig. 2–7). Pull the

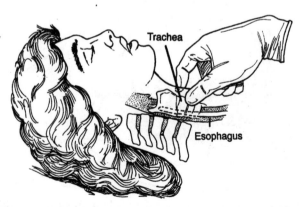

Figure 2–6. The Sellick maneuver. The thumb and index finger press down on the cricoid cartilage, compressing the esophagus against the spine.

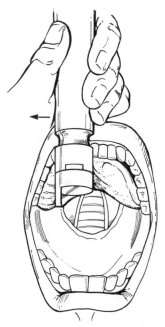

Figure 2–7. Inserting the laryngoscope in the right corner of the mouth pushes the tongue out of the way. This allows visualization of the cords and passage of the endotracheal tube.

handle of the laryngoscope in the direction that it points (90° to the blade). Avoid cocking the handle back, which can break the teeth. Pass the endotracheal tube only after you see the true vocal cords or glottic aperture. Watch the tube go through the cords until the black stripe on the distal end of the endotracheal tube has passed all the way through the cords. If you see the glottis but cannot advance the tube, have your assistant reduce the cricoid pressure. You may find Magil forceps helpful in this situation. Confirm tube placement by the following methods:

a. Presence of breath sounds over both lungs (especially over the left axilla)
b. Improved oxygenation
c. Increasing end-tidal CO_2 (if available)

 d. Fogging of the tube
 e. Chest x-ray

Free aspiration of > 10 to 20 mL of air from the end of the endotracheal tube is a simple method of verifying placement in the trachea. If you're not sure whether the tube is correctly placed, pull it out and make a second attempt! After inflating the endotracheal tube cuff with 10 mL of air, release cricoid pressure and secure the tube with tape or umbilical cord. The end of the endotracheal tube should then be connected to a BVM or ventilator. At this point, consider giving additional sedation or paralysis as indicated. Oxygen saturation should be monitored by pulse oximetry during the procedure. Desaturation should be avoided. If you are unable to intubate, stop and manually ventilate the patient with a BVM before reattempting intubation.

Although it is important to be familiar with all the medications used in RSI (Table 2–1), it is easiest to remember one standard formula that is effective in most cases:

1. Preoxygenate.
2. Prepare all equipment.
3. Pretreat with vecuronium (defasciculating dose = 1 mg).
4. Induce with etomidate 0.3 mg/kg IVP (rapid, short-acting, minimal myocardial and respiratory depression).
5. Paralyze with succinylcholine 1.5 mg/kg IVP (rapid, short-acting).
6. Intubate and confirm tube placement.

Modification of the standard sequence of RSI should be made in the following conditions:

- **Increased ICP:** Pretreat with lidocaine and fentanyl (3 µg/kg IVP) to blunt the increase in ICP with laryngoscopy and intubation. Consider induction with thiopental in isolated head injuries.
- **Status asthmaticus:** Use ketamine (1 mg/kg IVP), which has direct bronchodilatory effects and leads to release of catecholamines, for induction.
- **Congestive heart failure (CHF):** Avoid myocardial depressants, such as thiopental and succinylcholine. Etomidate and vecuronium are good alternatives.
- **Status epilepticus:** Induce with thiopental, which suppresses epileptogenic foci and increases the seizure threshold.

Table 2-1. DRUGS USED IN RAPID SEQUENCE INTUBATION

Medication	Dose (mg/kg)	Onset (min)	Duration (min)	Comments
Etomidate	0.2–0.3	1	4–10	Nausea, vomiting, myoclonus, adrenal suppression, cardiac depression; agent of choice in trauma and CHF
Thiopental	3.0–5.0	1	10–30	Hypotension, histamine release; decreases ICP
Midazolam	0.1–0.2	1	30–80	Minimal adverse effects; can be given IM
Ketamine	1.0	1	15–30	Emergent hallucinations, increased BP, bronchodilation
Propofol	1.0–2.0	10–15 secs	6–10	Hypotension
Succinylcholine	1.5	<1	6–12	Bradycardia, hyperkalemia, masseter muscle spasm, malignant hyperthermia, increased ICP; contraindicated in penetrating eye injuries
Vecuronium	0.1–0.2	1–2	40–60	Minimal adverse effects
Pancuronium	0.05–0.10	3	40–60	Lower dosage in renal failure; vagolytic
Mevicurium	0.15–0.3	1–2	12–30	Releases histamine
Rocuronium	0.6–1.0	1	30–60	Few cardiovascular events; safe in chronic renal failure
Rapacuronium	1.5	<1	15–25	Responsive to reversal with neostygmine; rarely, bronchospasm

BP = blood pressure; CHF = congestive heart failure; ICP = intracranial pressure; IM = intramuscularly.

- **Blunt multiple trauma:** Patients often are hypotensive; therefore, etomidate, which causes minimal myocardial depression, is the preferred induction agent. *Be aware that as you intubate a hypovolemic patient and ventilate with positive-pressure breathing, right ventricular filling may be impeded, resulting in a decrease in the systemic blood pressure (BP). Treat this with fluids and minimization of high airway pressures, continuing sedation, or paralysis as required.*

BREATHING

Assessment

After ensuring an open airway, assess whether the patient is breathing adequately. Look for signs of chest wall movement and symmetry. Feel and listen for air movement. Auscultate with a stethoscope for bilateral breath sounds and for sounds heard over the stomach. The patient in respiratory failure may be tachypnic, cyanotic, speechless, or lethargic. Paradoxical abdominal breathing (inward abdominal movement with inspiration), as well as suprasternal, subcostal, and intercostal retractions, all are evidence of respiratory distress. Look for signs of a tension pneumothorax (tracheal deviation away from the side of decreased breath sounds, jugular venous distention). If the patient is not breathing adequately, assist ventilation with a BVM or a ventilator.

Ventilators

Pressure-cycled respirators usually are used in infants weighing less than 10 kg, whereas volume-cycled respirators are used in larger patients.

Initial ventilator settings may be estimated with the following formulas:

1. Tidal volume (TV): 10 to 20 mL/kg.
2. Respiratory rate (RR): 12 to 16 breaths per minute (faster in a patient with suspected increased ICP).
3. FIO_2: Start with 100%; then adjust to maintain an O_2 saturation > 90%.

If the patient remains hypoxic despite 100% O_2, check for pneumothorax. If none exists, consider adding positive end-expiratory pressure (PEEP) in increments of 2 cm

H_2O. ABGs should be drawn within 10 to 15 minutes to en-sure proper ventilation and oxygenation.

Ventilating the Severely Tight Asthmatic

Sometimes it is technically difficult to ventilate the pa-tient with severe bronchospasm. Low tidal volumes should be used, and the RR should be adjusted to maintain ade-quate oxygenation ($PaO_2 > 60$). Hyperventilation should be avoided, however, because it can cause dangerously high airway pressures, with resultant barotrauma. High levels of CO_2 may need to be tolerated (permissive hyper-capnea). Also, the inspiratory-to-expiratory ratio should be adjusted for a prolonged expiratory phase.

Interpretation of Arterial Blood Gases

It is beyond the scope of this book to review ABG analy-sis in detail, so we will provide only an overview. ABGs measure the following parameters:

1. **$PaCO_2$:** This is a direct measure of ventilation. A $PaCO_2$ <35 means that the patient is hyperventilating. A $PaCO_2$ >45 means that the patient is hypoventilating. Note that some patients with chronic obstructive pulmonary disease chronically retain CO_2, and in these patients, the pH should be used to assess ventilation.
2. **PaO_2:** This is a measure of the adequacy of oxygenation. Calculating the alveolar-arterial oxygen gradient (A-a gradient) helps to sort out the various causes of hypox-emia. For example, in a patient breathing room air at sea level, the alveolar PO_2 may be estimated by sub-tracting the $PaCO_2$ from 145:

$$A\text{-a gradient} = (145 - PaCO_2) - PaO_2$$

The A-a gradient is then calculated by subtracting the PaO_2 from the **PAO_2.** Hypoxia with a normal A-a gradi-ent (10–15) is rare and is caused by hypoventilation or a low alveolar FIO_2. Hypoxia with an increased A-a gra-dient is more common, usually due to mismatched ventilation-perfusion ($\dot{V}/\dot{Q}$ mismatch). Arteriovenous shunting or a diffusion barrier are other causes of hy-poxemia with an increased A-a gradient. Failure of the hypoxia to respond to 100% O_2 suggests a right-left shunt.

3. **pH:** This defines the acid-base balance. Many disturbances are mixed. In pure acid-base disturbances, the relationships among pH, $PaCO_2$, and HCO_3 can be estimated using the following formulas:
   a. In metabolic acidosis, the $PaCO_2$ should equal 1.5 (HCO_3) + 8.
   b. In metabolic alkalosis, the $PaCO_2$ should equal 0.9 (HCO_3).
   c. In respiratory acidosis, the HCO_3 should increase by 1 mEq/L for every 10 mm Hg increase in $PaCO_2$.
   d. In respiratory alkalosis, the HCO_3 should fall 2 mEq/L for every 10 mm Hg decrease in $PaCO_2$.

If the changes in $PaCO_2$ or HCO_3 differ significantly from the expected compensatory changes, a mixed acid-base disturbance should be suspected.

Figures 2–8 and 2–9 present a useful approach to the differential diagnosis of acid-base disturbances.

CIRCULATION AND SHOCK

The circulatory system is composed of a *pump* (the heart), *fluid* (the blood), and a system of *tubes* (blood vessels). Its purpose is to supply vital nutrients (e.g., oxygen, glucose) to the tissues and to return waste products (e.g., carbon dioxide) for elimination. *Shock* is defined as a state

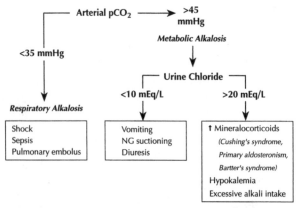

Figure 2–8. The differential diagnosis of alkalemia.

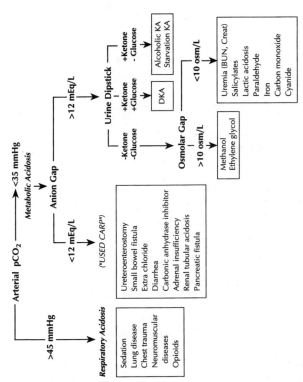

Figure 2–9. The differential diagnosis of acidemia.

of circulatory insufficiency, whereby perfusion is inadequate to meet the metabolic needs of the cells. Classification of the stages of shock is presented in Chapter 3.

The major pitfalls in shock management are failure to recognize circulatory insufficiency in its earlier states, awaiting a drop in the arterial BP before diagnosing shock, and insufficient fluid resuscitation. **PEARL: Remember that children's blood pressure may not drop until a cardiopulmonary arrest.**

Cause of Shock

Ultimately, shock management requires recognition and correction of the underlying cause. The following are the more common causes of shock seen in the ED according to mechanism:

- **Hypovolemic shock** (failure of fluids) is the most common cause of shock seen in the trauma patient and is usually due to blood loss. Other causes of hypovolemic shock include diarrhea, vomiting, and overzealous diuresis. See Table 3–1 for a classification of hypovolemic shock.
- **Cardiogenic shock** (pump failure) is due to abnormalities of chronotropy (both rapid and slow heart rates) or inotropy (systolic or diastolic myocardial dysfunction).
- **Distributive shock** (failure of tubes) is due to redistribution of the fluids within the circulatory system, resulting in inadequate flow. This type of shock includes septic, neurogenic, and anaphylactic shock.

Assessment of Shock

Shock is characterized by a low flow state. An extreme state of shock is seen in cases of cardiac or traumatic arrest, where there is no flow at all. **PEARL: Do not rely on a blood pressure reading alone to determine or to assess for shock; assess tissue perfusion.** Assess tissue perfusion by examining the following clinical parameters:

- **Pulse:** After assessing the airway and breathing, check for a pulse. The peripheral pulse usually is lost when the systemic arterial BP falls below 70 to 80 mm Hg; therefore, start by assessing a central pulse at the carotid or femoral arteries. If a central pulse is palpated, check a peripheral pulse for the following characteristics.

- Is it rapid? (You don't have to count the heart rate to know that it is too fast!)
- Is it weak and thready?

- **Central nervous system (CNS):** One of the earliest signs of shock is agitation. As the systemic arterial BP falls below 80 mm Hg, the patient becomes confused and ultimately loses consciousness.
- **Skin:** As blood is shunted away from the skin to preserve cerebral and cardiac circulation, the skin becomes cool and clammy. In the past, much emphasis was placed on capillary refill as a good indicator of peripheral perfusion. More recent studies, however, have failed to validate its usefulness.
- **Cardiac:** In cases of severe shock, especially in patients with underlying coronary artery disease, the myocardium can become ischemic; the patient complains of chest pain or shortness of breath and may develop a tachycardia.
- **Systemic BP:** Because of compensatory mechanisms (mainly sympathetic stimulation), supine BP usually is maintained until more than 25% to 30% of the blood volume is lost. Also remember that although a BP of 120/80 mm Hg often is felt to be normal, BPs vary widely. Therefore, *do not rely on BP measurement to estimate the adequacy of circulation.*
- **Renal:** Normal urine output is approximately 30 to 50 mL/h (1 mL/kg per hour in children). Decreased urinary output is an early sign of shock, so accurate assessment of urinary output is one of the cornerstones of shock evaluation and management.
- **pH:** The presence of metabolic acidosis suggests severe hypoperfusion and advanced shock.

DYSRHYTHMIAS

A detailed description of the various dysrhythmias is beyond the scope of this book; rather, we present a simplified approach to the unstable patient with an arrhythmia. Generally, to manage the unstable patient, you should be able to answer the following questions.

- Is there a pulse?
- What is the heart rate?
- Is the rhythm organized?

Figure 2–10 presents a simple approach to managing dysrhythmias in the unstable patient.

ARRESTS AND RESUSCITATIONS

Most patients who come into the ED *in extremis* are brought in by EMS. Don't miss this opportunity to obtain vital information concerning the patient's present and past illnesses. Often, the patient is brought in without family members or friends, and this might be your only chance to obtain pertinent information concerning the patient. All the relevant information should be obtained briefly from the EMS crew while the patient is being wheeled into the room and transferred from the stretcher to the bed. Also don't forget that many EDs have telemetry capabilities and serve as EMS base stations; much vital information can be obtained even before the patient arrives at the ED.

The following information should be obtained from prehospital personnel before their departure from the ED:

- The length of time that the patient has been unresponsive (or the time the patient was found).
- Presence and timing of bystander cardiopulmonary resuscitation (CPR).
- Length of time until arrival of EMS and initiation of CPR.
- Initial rhythm and vital signs.
- Therapy given at the scene and en route, and the patient's response.
- Brief description of the scene of arrest (e.g., evidence of trauma, overdose).
- Evidence and estimation of external blood loss.
- Medical history, medications, and allergies, if known.
- Presence of "do not resuscitate" (DNR) orders, advance directives, health care proxy, or a living will.

On learning about the imminent arrival of a patient *in extremis*, the following preparations will expedite the care of the patient on arrival:

1. Prepare an airway station—suction apparatus, laryngoscopy, endotracheal tubes, BVM, and O_2.

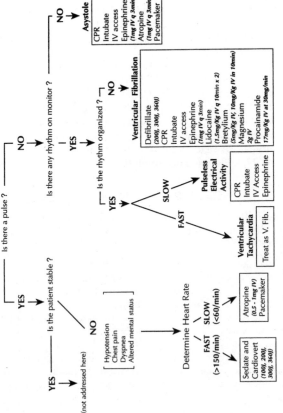

Figure 2–10. Approach to dysrhythmias.

2. Prepare IV access and fluids—large-bore (#14- or #16-gauge) angiocatheters and several bags of normal saline (NS) solution with tubing. Also, have syringes, needles, and lab tubes available.
3. Notify backup teams as needed and required by the nature of the case (e.g., surgeons, anesthesiologists, respiratory therapists, or pediatricians).
4. Determine the team leader and delegate responsibilities to the team members, such as IV access, airway management, defibrillation, medication administration, and documentation.
5. Dress for the occasion. Resuscitations, whether medical or traumatic, can be very messy (e.g., blood, vomitus). Put on gloves, mask, goggles or face shield, water-resistant gown, and shoe covers before the patient's arrival.

Advanced cardiac life support (ACLS) guidelines and treatment protocols appear in Appendix A. You are strongly encouraged to read the original recommendations in the August 22, 2000 issue of *Circulation*.

GENERAL RECOMMENDATIONS

The following general recommendations can help you avoid the more common mistakes and pitfalls in ED resuscitations:

1. Turn chaos into control by establishing yourself as the team leader and discourage unnecessary noises and distractions. (Remember, however, that you will need help: You can't do everything yourself.)
2. Don't forget to apply "quick look" paddles first before establishing IVs, performing endotracheal intubation, and so on.
3. If the patient is in ventricular fibrillation, apply three defibrillations as required, in rapid succession. Do not waste time checking for a pulse between *initial* defibrillations.
4. Initially, peripheral IV access should be obtained, but central venous access should be established as soon as practical because central drug administration has been shown to be more effective than peripheral administration. In children, if IV access is not obtained within 60 seconds, intraosseous access should be performed at the midanterior tibia (Fig. 2–11).

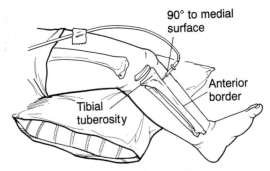

Figure 2–11. Intraosseous cannulation technique.

5. Don't forget to defibrillate the patient 30 to 60 seconds after each drug is administered for ventricular fibrillation. After drug administration, flush the line with 10 to 20 mL NS to facilitate its distribution.
6. Continuously reassess the patient for the presence of a pulse and spontaneous respirations. Endotracheal tube placement and the patient's color also should be reevaluated.
7. Don't forget to give magnesium 2 g IV for resistant ventricular fibrillation. Amiodarone 150 to 300 mg IV may also be attempted.
8. Transcutaneous pacing in patients with bradycardia or asystole, when readily available, is extremely useful.
9. If pulseless electrical activity is present, attempt to rule out underlying conditions, such as:
    a. Hypovolemia (give a fluid bolus)
    b. Tension pneumothorax (perform bilateral needle thoracostomies)
    c. Pericardial tamponade (perform pericardiocentesis)
    d. Acidosis (correct ventilation and administer bicarbonate for a pH < 7.1)
    e. Hyperkalemia (give calcium chloride and bicarbonate)

3
CHAPTER

Trauma

▶ Rapid transport of all trauma patients to the nearest trauma center is imperative.
▶ All multiple-trauma patients should be immobilized with a stiff collar and backboard and receive 100% oxygen with a nonrebreather mask.
▶ Large-bore IV access should be established en route to the hospital, if possible, to minimize the amount of time spent at the scene.
▶ Rapid infusion of crystalloids should be considered in all hemodynamically unstable patients.

GENERAL PRINCIPLES

In no other situation is it more important to perform a rapid and thorough assessment than in the multiply injured patient. Your goal is to identify and initiate management for those salvageable injuries that can cause death (if unrecognized) during the first "golden hour." Although the assessment and management of the multiply injured patient is presented here in a sequential manner in order of priority, in the clinical setting, multiple steps should be addressed simultaneously.

History

Trauma can be divided into two major types: *blunt* and *penetrating*. Blunt trauma is often multiple and occult, whereas penetrating trauma is more limited and readily apparent. Therefore, patients with blunt trauma have greater mortality and morbidity secondary to a delay in diagnosis.

Ascertaining the mechanism of initial trauma can help you to predict the types and severity of resulting injuries. Each type of trauma injury is associated with a distinct set of circumstances. Therefore, one must gather all of the following relevant information:

- **Motor vehicle accidents:** What was the direction of impact; appearance of vehicle (body, windshield, steering wheel, and column); use of restraining devices, seat belts, and/or air bags; and estimated speed at impact (remember energy equals mass times velocity squared)? Ejection of the patient from the vehicle or the death of another passenger significantly increases the likelihood that the patient has serious injuries. Also, try to estimate the degree of external blood loss at the scene.
- **Falls:** From what height and onto what type of surface did the patient fall?
- **Penetrating trauma:** Where was the patient injured? What weapon was used? What was the estimated distance of the patient from the weapon? What was the velocity and caliber of the bullet?

Other important information that should be considered in your evaluation includes damage to structures surrounding the trauma victim at the scene, extrication problems, injuries suffered by others in the same event, events preceding the injury, recent alcohol or drug use, and last oral intake of food or beverage. Also obtain a history of prior illnesses, surgeries, medications, immunizations, and allergies.

Patient management consists of a rapid primary evaluation, resuscitation of vital functions, a more detailed secondary evaluation, and finally, the initiation of definitive care.

THE PRIMARY SURVEY: ASSESSMENT OF THE ABCDEs

During the initial stage of patient evaluation and assessment (the primary survey), you must recognize life-threatening conditions and initiate management simultaneously. Once a problem is identified, it must be addressed before proceeding to the next stage. The mnemonic ABCDE will help you to remember the sequence of patient evaluation during the primary survey: A, airway; B, breathing; C, circulation; D, disability; E, exposure.

Airway and Cervical Spine

Cervical spine (C-spine) injuries are present in approximately 1% to 2% of all blunt trauma patients and in 5% to 10% of patients with head trauma. **PEARL: It is safest always to assume a C-spine fracture is present.** Excessive motion of the unstable C-spine (both hyperextension and hyperflexion) can cause further neurologic damage.

Rapidly assess the upper airway for obstruction (see Chapter 2). Use the chin lift and/or jaw thrust to establish airway patency. Look in the mouth for foreign bodies, debris, and vomitus. If the airway is compromised, rapid-sequence induction (RSI) with in-line C-spine immobilization is the preferred method of airway control.

The following is a summary of RSI in the patient with trauma:

1. **Preoxygenate** with 100% O_2.
2. **Pretreat** with vecuronium (0.01 mg/kg IVP), lidocaine (1.5 mg/kg IVP), and fentanyl (3 to 5 μg/ kg JV).
3. **Induce** with etomidate (0.3 mg/kg IVP, with multiple injuries) or thiopental (3 to 5 mg/kg IVP in isolated head injuries).
4. **Paralyze** with succinylcholine (1.5 mg/kg IV). Children under age 5 should be pretreated with atropine 0.01 mg/kg IV.
5. **Perform orotracheal intubation** with C-spine immobilization.

For a more detailed discussion of RSI, refer to Chapter 2.

If you are unable to intubate the patient because of obstructive lesions, you must perform needle or surgical cricothyroidotomy through the cricothyroid membrane. You can find this membrane by locating the suprasternal notch and advancing your finger cephalad in the midline. The first hard cartilaginous structure you encounter is the cricoid cartilage. The soft cricothyroid membrane is immediately above this and below the thyroid cartilage (the "Adam's apple," Fig. 3–1).

Needle cricothyroidotomy is performed by inserting a large-bore angiocatheter attached to a 10-mL syringe

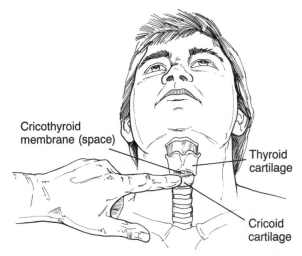

Figure 3–1. Cricothyroid membrane anatomy.

through this membrane at a 45° angle in the caudal direction. Aspirating for air while advancing can help prevent cannulation of the esophagus or the soft tissues. The hub of the angiocatheter should be connected to a 3-mm endotracheal tube adapter or to a 3-mL syringe and 7.5-mm adapter, which enables ventilation with a BVM (Fig. 3–2). Use of a jet insufflator at a pressure of 50 pounds per square inch (psi), however, is the most effective method to ensure adequate oxygenation and ventilation. Use this method only as a temporizing agent because it can result in hypercarbia after 30 minutes.

Surgical cricothyroidotomy is the definitive surgical airway. A midline superficial vertical incision is made between the suprasternal notch and the thyroid cartilage. After the cricothyroid membrane is identified, a horizontal incision is made through it by gently puncturing it with the tip of a #11 blade. This opening then is enlarged with a surgical clamp, and a 6-mm endotracheal tube (or specialized tracheostomy tube) is inserted between the spread ends of the clamp (Fig. 3–3). Avoid surgical cricothyroidotomy in children younger than 8 years old because of their small airways.

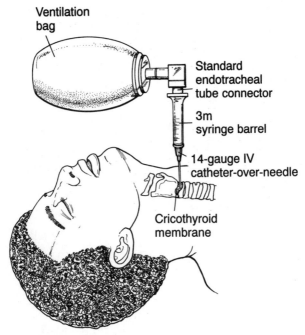

Figure 3–2. Needle cricothyroidotomy.

Breathing

During this stage, attempt to identify the three traumatic conditions that most often severely compromise ventilation: (1) tension pneumothorax, (2) open pneumothorax, and (3) large flail chests with an underlying pulmonary contusion. Examine the chest and assess for adequacy of air exchange:

- Is the chest wall moving?
- Is the movement symmetric?
- Are there any obvious injuries (e.g., open wounds, contusions, abrasions)?
- Auscultate below the armpits bilaterally for the presence of breath sounds.
- Is the trachea midline?
- Is there jugular venous distention?
- Is there paradoxic motion of a flail segment of the chest?

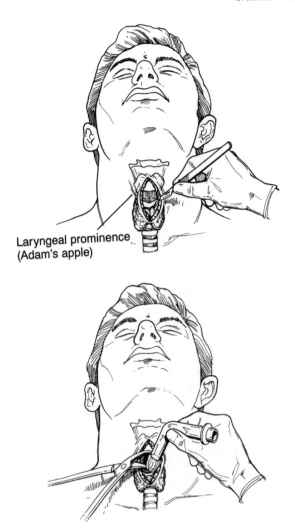

Laryngeal prominence
(Adam's apple)

Figure 3–3. Surgical cricothyroidotomy.

If you suspect a tension pneumothorax (i.e., respiratory distress, absent breath sounds, deviated trachea and mediastinum, elevated central venous pressure, and poor peripheral perfusion), insert a #18- or #16-gauge angiocatheter attached to a fluid-filled syringe in the second intercostal space at the midclavicular line. The appearance of air bubbles in the fluid-filled syringe both confirms and decompresses a pneumothorax (remember that the patient will need a more definitive chest tube placed after you complete your primary survey). If you find an open chest wound, an occlusive dressing should be placed immediately. If one is already in place or if on placing an occlusive dressing the patient's respiratory status suddenly deteriorates, remove the occlusive dressing and insert a chest tube before reapplying an occlusive dressing.

All trauma patients should receive supplemental 100% O_2 via a nonrebreather mask or a BVM.

Circulation

Significant external bleeding should be identified and controlled during the primary survey by direct manual pressure on the wound. Do not blindly insert surgical clamps in wounds in an attempt to stop bleeding. Peripheral perfusion is assessed by examining the patient's level of consciousness, pulse, BP, skin, urine output, and ABGs (for a detailed discussion of assessing tissue perfusion, see Chapter 2).

Hemorrhagic shock secondary to acute blood loss is the most common cause of shock in trauma patients. Other causes of shock should always be considered, however, especially if the patient is not responding to treatment. *Cardiogenic shock* may be due to underlying cardiac disease or may be the result of a cardiac contusion or pericardial tamponade. *Neurogenic shock* should be considered in patients with relative bradycardia and warm skin. *Hypovolemic shock* is divided into four stages of increasing severity based on the degree of blood loss. Table 3–1 is a useful classification of shock based on the percentage of volume lost, the average blood loss, and the presence of clinical parameters.

Early recognition of the shock state, aggressive fluid management, and identification and correction of the underlying cause are the cornerstones of management. In many trauma patients, this means getting them to the operating room as soon as possible. **PEARL: Don't delay the transport of an unstable patient to the operating room to complete physical, radiologic, or lab assessment (all may be completed in the operating room).**

Table 3–1. CLASSIFICATION OF STAGES OF HYPOVOLEMIC SHOCK

Class	Blood Loss	Physical Examination Findings	Therapy
I	15% (750 mL)	Normal	Ringer's lactate, normal saline
II	15%–30% (750–1500 mL)	Normal BP, tachycardia, anxious	Ringer's lactate, normal saline
III	30%–40% (1500–2000 mL)	May be hypotensive, tachycardia, confused/combative, metabolic acidosis	Ringer's lactate, normal saline *plus* Packed red blood cells (PRBCs)
IV Profound shock	> 40% (> 2000 mL)	Obvious hypotension, tachycardia, coma	Ringer's lactate, normal saline *plus* PRBCs

Intravenous Access

Intravenous access must be established as soon as possible with at least two large-bore peripheral IVs (#14- or #16-gauge angiocatheters). Central venous catheters are not part of the initial resuscitation unless no other access is available. They may play an important diagnostic and monitoring role later in the management, but they are rarely required during the primary survey.

The following are sites for IV access *in order of preference* (remember that this is not the time to save the "best" veins for last to demonstrate your skills as a phlebotomist):

1. **Antecubital veins,** which usually are easy to visualize or palpate.
2. **Other peripheral upper-extremity veins** in the forearm or hand. The cephalic vein, located over the lateral radial aspect of the wrist, is often a good choice.
3. **Saphenous venous cutdown.** Perform a 2-cm horizontal incision, 1 cm anterior and 1 cm proximal to the medial malleolus at the ankle. Isolate the greater saphenous vein by blunt dissection with a curved hemostat, and cannulate with a large-bore angiocatheter (Fig. 3–4).
4. **The femoral vein,** which is located medial to the femoral artery distal to the inguinal ligament. If no pulse is palpable, insert the needle distal to the inguinal ligament one finger breadth medial to the halfway point between the anterior superior iliac spine and the pubic tubercle (Fig. 3–5). An 8F catheter should be introduced into the vein over a wire. This may be faster and easier than a saphenous venous cutdown.
5. **Subclavian or internal jugular vein,** whichever you are more comfortable with. Use an 8F short catheter. Beside ultrasound, using a 7.5 MHz transducer may help locate the veins in different situations.

Fluids

Although the issue of crystalloids versus colloids is controversial, crystalloids should be the initial choice in shock. **PEARL: Don't be afraid to push fluids in patients with head or spinal cord injuries who are hemodynamically unstable.** Either normal saline (NS) or lactated Ringer's solution may be used. As a rule, three times as much crystalloids are required to replace the loss of a given amount of blood. Begin by giving a 2-liter fluid bolus as rapidly as possible

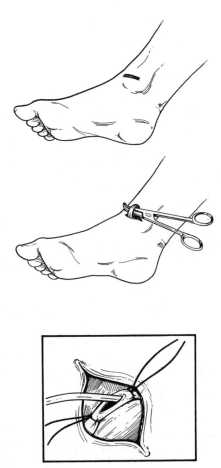

Figure 3–4. Saphenous venous cutdown.

(rapid infusion pumps are available in some emergency departments). Further fluid management is determined by the response to this initial fluid challenge. **PEARL: Give blood to hemodynamically unstable patients not responding to crystalloids.** If the patient remains hypotensive, give blood. Although type-specific blood is preferable (usually available within 10 minutes), type O-negative blood should be given if the patient is hemodynamically unstable.

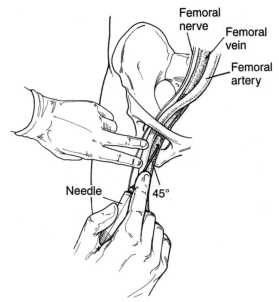

Figure 3–5. Femoral vein cannulation.

Blood is most often given as packed red blood cells (PRBCs). Generally, give 2 U of fresh frozen plasma for every 6 U of PRBCs transfused. With very rapid infusion of blood, both platelets and calcium chloride may be required. *Note that blood products must be diluted with NS, not lactated Ringer's solution.* **PEARL: Avoid overly aggressive fluid resuscitation in the hemodynamically stable patient with head or spinal cord injuries.**

Disability

During the primary survey, a brief neurologic evaluation, including level of consciousness and a pupil examination, should be performed:

1. The patient's level of consciousness can be described using the AVPU method:

   A alert
   V responds to *vocal* stimuli

P responds to *painful* stimuli (pain should be applied above the clavicles, such as supraorbital pressure)

U unresponsive to all stimuli

The GCS is rarely necessary in the primary survey; it is used during the secondary survey. If the patient is to be intubated and paralyzed, however, rapid GCS assessment is essential for the neurosurgeon. Often it is enough to say, "Open your eyes," and note the response to noxious stimuli, such as IV attempts.

2. **Pupils:** Look at the pupils. Note their size. Are they equal? Do they react to light? Pupillary inequality (anisocoria) or unresponsiveness may be a sign of increased intracranial pressure (ICP), resulting in uncal herniation and pressure on the third cranial nerve nucleus on the side of the larger pupil. Note that in the normal population, 10% to 15% of people have anisocoria in which the pupils do respond to light.

Exposure

Completely undress the patient and remove all garments and jewelry. Now is not the time to be modest. All nooks and crannies must be assessed. It is important to log roll the patient while maintaining C-spine immobilization to examine the back and buttock areas. After completing your assessment, cover the patient with a warm blanket. It is easier to prevent hypothermia than to treat the resulting complications. **PEARL: Always get a rectal temperature. Hypothermia should be avoided and aggressively managed.**

Monitoring

All patients in shock should be connected to a cardiac monitor and pulse oximetry. Place an automated BP monitor or an arterial line. If the patient remains hypotensive, consider inserting a central venous pressure catheter to assess for elevated right-sided pressures that may be caused by pericardial tamponade or for very low pressures that require more aggressive fluid or blood resuscitation.

RESUSCITATION

Although presented separately, resuscitative efforts should be instituted while the primary and secondary surveys are being performed.

The following elements should be part of the resuscitation of all trauma patients:

- **O_2:** All patients should receive supplemental O_2 via a nonrebreather mask or a BVM.
- **IV access:** All patients should have at least two peripheral large-bore IVs established, as described previously in this chapter under IV Access (i.e., in patients in hypovolemic shock). When inserting an IV, blood should be drawn immediately for type and cross-match as well as for a baseline complete blood count (CBC), chemistry, and amylase. Seriously injured patients should have a spun hematocrit (for more details on how to spin a "crit," see Chapter 11). If you insert an angiocatheter and have difficulty obtaining the required amount of blood, draw blood from the femoral artery to avoid wasting precious time.
- **Urinary output:** Output should be monitored after an indwelling urethral catheter is placed. Attempts should be made first to obtain a spontaneously voided urine because urethral catheterization can cause injury and some bleeding. **PEARL: Always examine the genitalia and perform a rectal examination before inserting a urethral catheter.** Contraindications to urinary catheterization include blood at the external meatus, perineal or scrotal hematoma, and a high-riding or nonpalpable prostate. If a urinary catheter cannot be placed, the patient will need an emergent retrograde urethrogram.
- **Gastric catheters:** Gastric catheters should be considered at this point. Aspiration of blood suggests gastrointestinal injury. Emptying the stomach also reduces the risk of aspiration and relieves pressure on the diaphragm that can limit adequate ventilation. In cases of significant nasal trauma or suspected skull fracture, an orogastric tube should be placed (because of the risk of a nasal approach leading to intracranial intubation). Early placement of a gastric catheter also enables administration of oral contrast when an abdominal computed tomographic (CT) scan is required.
- **Radiologic trauma screen:** A screen should be obtained, including a cross-table lateral view of the neck, a supine anteroposterior view of the chest, and a pelvic view. It is easiest to film all three areas in rapid succession before having the technician develop the

films. All other x-rays should be performed after stabilization and performance of a more detailed secondary survey.

THE SECONDARY SURVEY

The secondary survey consists of a thorough head-to-toe evaluation of the patient including assessment of vital signs. **PEARL: Continually reassess the patient's vital signs, airway, and endotracheal tube placement.** This survey must not be performed before initial patient stabilization. A complete description of the secondary survey can be found in the ATLS manual. Several often-neglected areas are highlighted.

Head

- Paper clips bent in two can be used to create eyelid retractors when eye opening is difficult.
- Epistaxis (nosebleed) should be tamponaded with a nasal tampon.
- A nasal septal hematoma should be drained with a #18-gauge needle or a #11 blade (see Chapter 9).
- A hemotympanum is the most common clinical finding in basilar skull fractures.

Central Nervous System

The patient's level of consciousness, based on the GCS, should be assessed (Table 3–2). The neurologic status should be reassessed repeatedly (every 10 to 15 minutes) for signs of deterioration.

Increased ICP with herniation is suggested by the following signs and symptoms:

- GCS < 8
- Unequal pupils (anisocoria > 1 mm) in a patient with an altered mental status
- Cushing's triad (hypertension, bradycardia, and abnormal respirations)
- Deteriorating neurologic status
- Significant edema or midline shift visualized on a head CT scan
- Lateralizing neurologic signs

Table 3–2. THE GLASGOW COMA SCALE

1. Best Verbal Response

None	1
Incomprehensible sounds	2
Inappropriate words	3
Confused	4
Oriented	5

2. Eye Opening

None	1
To pain	2
To command	3
Spontaneously	4

3. Best Motor Response

None	1
Abnormal extension	2
Abnormal flexion	3
Withdrawal	4
Localizes	5
Obeys commands	6

Total Score	**3–15**

The following measures will help decrease ICP:

1. Elevate the head of the bed to 30° if shock has been corrected.
2. Intubate and hyperventilate the patient *down* to a $PaCO_2$ of approximately 30 mm Hg by ventilating the patient 20 times per minute (once the $PaCO_2$ drops below 30 mm Hg, significant cerebral vasoconstriction will occur and cause a decreased perfusion pressure that can cause more ischemic damage).
3. Give mannitol 1 g/kg IV rapidly (avoid in the hypotensive patient).
4. Sedate the patient; give morphine sulfate 0.1 mg/kg IV every hour.
5. Paralyze the patient; give vecuronium or pancuronium 0.1 mg/kg IV every hour.
6. Maintain normothermia. (If patient is febrile, give antipyretics.)

Indications for a head CT scan in the multiply injured patient include:

- Head injury with skull penetration
- Any alteration in the level of consciousness
- A clear history of substantial loss of consciousness with memory deficit
- Focal neurologic findings or lateralization on examination
- Recurrent vomiting
- Increasing headache

Any patient with significant signs or symptoms suggesting intracranial injury should be admitted for observation and possibly a second head CT scan in 24 hours, even if the initial CT scan is negative.

Maxillofacial Trauma

Palpate for areas of tenderness and instability. Grasp the upper teeth and assess for midface instability. Have the patient open and close his or her mouth and assess for malocclusion.

Cervical Spine

Radiographic evaluation of the C-spine should include a cross-table lateral film, an anterior-posterior film, and an open-mouth view (odontoid film). If despite normal plain films you still suspect injury, additional films or scans of the neck [e.g., oblique, flexion-extension, CT, or magnetic resonance imaging (MRI)] may be performed. All seven vertebrae, including the C7 to T1 alignment, must be visualized. To facilitate visualization of the lower vertebrae, pull down on the patient's arms while obtaining the cross-table lateral film. If either of the arms is injured, wrap a long sheet around the shoulder from front to back and apply traction in the direction of the feet. If you still cannot see all the cervical vertebrae, a "swimmer's" view is recommended.

No x-ray is indicated if all of the following criteria are fulfilled:

- The patient is alert.
- The patient is not intoxicated.
- There are no significant distracting injuries (i.e., an extremity fracture).

- There is no midline neck tenderness.
- The patient denies having any neck pain.

Remove the cervical collar and ask the patient to move his or her head. If the patient has severe pain or great difficulty, obtain films.

Chest

The presence of deformities, ecchymosis, subcutaneous emphysema, and unequal breath sounds can suggest significant thoracic pathology.

Distant heart sounds and distended neck veins can indicate cardiac tamponade (in the presence of hypovolemia, however, neck veins may not be distended). Indications for chest tube placement include:

- Penetrating trauma to the chest: Don't forget that high abdominal and flank injuries can also invade the pleural cavity.
- Hemothorax or pneumothorax.
- Subcutaneous emphysema and multiple rib fractures, especially if the patient is to be taken to the operating room and ventilated with positive pressure.

If a chest tube is indicated, insert a large chest tube (#34F) anterior to the midaxillary line at the level of the fifth intercostal space (at the level of the nipple in men or at the level of the inframammary fold in women) (Fig. 3–6A).

Prep and drape the chest at the site of insertion and, if time allows, locally anesthetize the skin and rib periosteum with 1% lidocaine. Make a horizontal 2- to 3-cm incision over the rib below the predetermined space. Then bluntly dissect through the subcutaneous tissues over the top of the rib, and carefully puncture the parietal pleura with the tip of a large clamp. Insert your finger into the incision, and to avoid further injury, perform a 360° sweep, feeling for organs (lungs, heart, liver, spleen) and adhesions before inserting the chest tube.

Because most trauma patients have a combined pneumothorax and hemothorax and are usually supine, direct your chest tube posteriorly, superiorly, and medially. Make sure all side holes are within the pleural cavity. Look for condensation in the chest tube. Do not let go of the tube until it is adequately secured with a #0 silk or mersilene suture and adhesive tape (Fig. 3–6C). The end of the chest

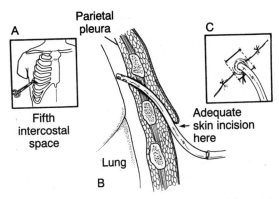

Figure 3–6. Chest tube placement. (A) Location of chest tube insertion. (B) Tunnel the tube through the subcutaneous tissue and above the rib superior to the site of insertion. (C) Secure the tube with a purse-string suture.

tube should be attached to an underwater seal apparatus and suction (-20 cm H_2O) or a Pleur-Evac. Verify tube placement and function by obtaining a stat chest x-ray.

Abdomen

Focus on determining whether an abdominal injury exists and surgical intervention is required. Frequent reassessments help you to identify any change in the patient's condition. The abdominal examination involves the following:

- **Inspection:** Are there any obvious penetrating injuries or evisceration of intra-abdominal organs (which usually are absolute indications for operative intervention)? (Some institutions are selective in cases of stab wounds.) Are there any significant abrasions or contusions indicating injury? Is the abdomen distended?
- **Palpation for areas of tenderness, rigidity, or masses:** Always perform a rectal examination for evidence of obvious rectal tears, pelvic fractures, or blood. Note the rectal tone and the position of the prostate gland.

Diagnostic Aids

The choice of abdominal CT, bedside ultrasonography, or peritoneal lavage for the evaluation of abdominal trauma is controversial and often institution-dependent. CT (with and without oral and IV contrast) gives the most specific anatomic information and allows assessment of the retroperitoneal space as well. If the patient is too unstable to be transferred to the CT scanner, however, peritoneal lavage or bedside ultrasound should be chosen. Performance of a rapid bedside ultrasound that allows early detection of intra-abdominal blood has become more acceptable and readily available in many institutions.

Indications for abdominal imaging include:

- Equivocal abdominal findings (e.g., in the presence of fractured ribs or lumbar spine fracture).
- The presence of head injury, intoxication, or paraplegia, which make the abdominal examination unreliable.
- Necessity of other lengthy evaluations or surgery (which precludes frequent reassessment).
- Unexplained hypotension. **PEARL: Never presume that hypotension is caused by a head injury.**

If you choose to perform a peritoneal lavage, we suggest that you use a semiopen technique with an incision through the skin and subcutaneous tissue before inserting a peritoneal dialysis catheter over a trocar. Have an assistant apply traction and elevate the abdominal wall with a pair of clamps. This will make using the peritoneal trocar easier and safer. Peritoneal lavage should be performed below the umbilicus in the midline (Fig. 3–7). Always decompress the stomach and bladder with a gastric tube and urinary catheter before performing lavage to avoid damage to these organs. Aspirate for blood or obvious enteric contents. If none is present, instill 1 liter of warm crystalloid (10 mL/kg in children) and then drain by gravity.

The following findings on peritoneal lavage often indicate the need for exploratory laparotomy:

- >5 mL of gross blood on aspiration
- Obvious enteric contents (food, feces)
- Appearance of peritoneal fluid in urinary catheter or chest tube
- 100,000 RBCs/mL of peritoneal lavage fluid

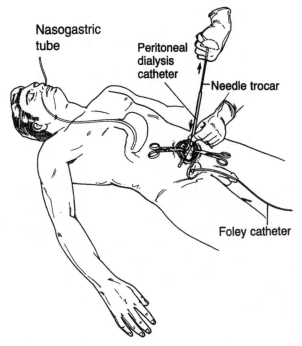

Figure 3–7. Peritoneal lavage. An assistant should place traction on the transversalis fascia and peritoneum.

- 500 white blood cells (WBCs)/mL of peritoneal lavage fluid
- Amylase > 175 U (controversial)

Surgery is also indicated in the unstable patient with evidence of intra-abdominal fluid on ultrasonography. Abdominal imaging should never be performed when early surgical intervention is clearly indicated, as in the hemodynamically unstable patient with evidence of abdominal trauma or in the patient with unequivocal peritoneal irritation.

Pelvis and Perineum

Urine should be obtained for a urine dipstick, which, if negative, reliably rules out hematuria. Remember that a positive dipstick may also be caused by hemoglobinuria (usually pink) or myoglobinuria (usually cola colored). Therefore, if the dipstick is positive, send urine for microscopic analysis to confirm the presence of hematuria. Isolated microhematuria in the hemodynamically stable patient does not require further workup. **PEARL: Perform a digital vaginal examination in female patients, looking for blood and evidence of a pelvic fracture.** Priapism in men suggests spinal cord injury.

Extremities

Inspect all extremities for swelling, ecchymosis, or obvious deformities. **PEARL: Palpate and document all extremity pulses.** All peripheral pulses should be assessed. If pulses are not palpable, try using a portable Doppler. Emergency arteriography should be considered in the presence of an arterial bleeder, an expanding hematoma, or a penetrating trauma in proximity to a major blood vessel.

Log roll the patient as a unit while immobilizing the head and neck, and inspect and palpate the thoracic and lumbar spine for areas of swelling, deformity, or tenderness. Don't forget to look between the buttocks for evidence of injury.

4

CHAPTER

Chest Pain

PREHOSPITAL CONSIDERATIONS

- ▶ Prehospital treatment for chest pain is usually aimed at cardiac ischemia.
- ▶ EMS personnel should obtain a rhythm strip and a 12-lead ECG, when possible. Their interpretation should be conveyed to the medical control operator.
- ▶ Usually, an IV line is started and the patient is placed on oxygen.
- ▶ Treatment for potential cardiac disease generally includes nitroglycerin and aspirin; if the cause is felt to be pulmonary (e.g., bronchospasm), bronchodilators may be given.
- ▶ The field diagnosis will need to be confirmed with in-hospital evaluation.

Chest pain is a very common chief complaint in most EDs. It can indicate disease ranging from the benign to the immediately fatal. In the evaluation of chest pain, the patient's history is vitally important. Physical examination and adjunctive tests can be helpful, but they often are normal, as in many cases of myocardial ischemia. Our concern is not to miss the diagnosis of serious cardiac, vascular, or respiratory disorders, such as myocardial infarction or unstable angina, new angina, pulmonary embolism (PE), or aortic dissection. **PEARL: All chest pain is serious until evaluated fully.**

HISTORY

Focus your questions on the character of the pain (e.g., sharp, dull), the time course of the pain (onset, duration), whether it is worsened by respiration (i.e., is the pain "pleuritic"), and what alleviating or aggravating factors there are. Pleuritic pain can indicate a noncardiac cause, such as costochondritis, pneumonia, or pneumothorax. Cardiac pain usually is not affected by the respiratory cycle, although pericarditis can give rise to pain that is aggravated by deep inspiration or a supine position. Also, ask about any recent chest trauma. Inquire about associated symptoms, such as cough and fever (think of pneumonia), or palpitations, nausea, shortness of breath, and diaphoresis (think of cardiac disease). Ask about cardiac risk factors: hypertension, diabetes, smoking, high cholesterol, sedentary lifestyle, or cardiac disease that developed in a first-degree relative younger than 50 years of age. Also, ask about recent use of cocaine, which can cause myocardial ischemia, often with an atypical presentation. **PEARL: Patients with chest pain who have used cocaine within the last 24 hours should be admitted to rule out cardiac ischemia or infarction.**

PHYSICAL EXAMINATION

Focus on the lungs and cardiovascular system. Listen for decreased breath sounds, wheezes, rubs, or rales. Murmurs or gallops may direct you to cardiac disease. Look for signs of congestive heart failure (CHF), such as peripheral edema, jugular venous distention, and hepatomegaly. **PEARL: The presence of cannon waves in the neck suggest AV dissociation, such as in ventricular tachycardia.** Examine the chest wall as well, looking for localized tenderness, ecchymosis, or rash (e.g., zoster). Reproducible chest wall tenderness does not exclude cardiac disease.

All patients with other than obviously benign chest pain should be placed on a cardiac monitor and pulse oximetry. To enable rapid drug administration in the event that a dysrhythmia should develop, IV access should be established before you conduct a comprehensive H&P.

ANCILLARY TESTS

Frequently, the tests of importance are the ECG and chest x-ray. In general, order an ECG for any patient with chest pain in whom you cannot absolutely exclude cardiac disease. Order a chest x-ray and pulse oximetry (or an ABG) for any patient with pulmonary signs or symptoms or in whom you suspect pulmonary disease. Patients with probable cardiac disease also should have an x-ray to look at heart size and evaluate for CHF. Every chest x-ray should be evaluated for the presence of a widened mediastinum (> 6 to 8 cm), suggesting aortic dissection, and pneumomediastinum, suggesting esophageal rupture.

Earlier and more sensitive and specific markers of myocardial injury [such as CPK-MB (creatine kinase MB fraction), myoglobin, and troponin I] are playing a more crucial role in the early decision-making process in the ED. When the results of such tests are readily available, a single negative test should never dissuade you from admitting a patient with a history that suggests myocardial ischemia. Some EDs have stress testing, sophisticated nuclear perfusion, or echocardiographic testing available, allowing discharge of low-risk patients with chest pain.

DIFFERENTIAL DIAGNOSIS

Certain causes of chest pain are so potentially dangerous that you must consider and exclude them for every patient with this complaint. Often, these problems have characteristic H&P findings, and the summary that follows should help you in sorting these out. Table 4–1 also includes some key points.

Aortic Dissection

Classically, patients with aortic dissection describe their pain as a sudden tearing, located in the mid or left chest or in the upper back. They often have a history of hypertension or have used drugs (e.g., cocaine) that can cause hypertension. Marfan syndrome predisposes patients to aortic dissection and should be considered in patients with marfanoid physical signs and symptoms (e.g., abnormally long extremities, especially fingers, lax joints, chest wall deformities, and other skeletal deformities).

Depending on which arteries have been disrupted by the dissection, patients may have neurologic deficits or unequal pulses or BPs in the extremities. If the dissection has compromised the coronary circulation, they can have the

Table 4–1. DIFFERENTIAL DIAGNOSIS OF CHEST PAIN

Etiology	Onset/Course	Typical Quality	Location/Radiation	Exacerbating Factors
Angina	Rapid/brief	Pressure	Chest, neck, arms	Exertion, stress
Myocardial infarction	Rapid/> 30 min	Pressure	Chest, neck, arms	Stress or none
Aortic dissection	Sudden/severe	Tearing	Chest and back	Hypertension
Pulmonary embolism	Sudden	Sharp, pleuritic	Chest, back	Deep breath, cough
Esophageal rupture	Sudden/severe	Sharp, burning	Chest, throat, back	Swallowing, vomiting
Pericarditis	Gradual	Sharp, pleuritic	Precordium	Supine position
Musculoskeletal	Variable	Sharp, dull	Localized	Movement

signs and symptoms of myocardial ischemia or infarction. The aortic valve can be damaged, leading to aortic regurgitation. The valve may be wide open so that there may not be a murmur. The dissection can also rupture into the pericardium, causing cardiac tamponade.

If you suspect dissection, the initial treatment is to lower the BP with IV nitroprusside (0.5 to 10.0 µg/kg per minute) and beta-blockers (labetolol IV in incremental boluses starting at 20 to 40 mg), or with trimethaphan IV (1 to 4 mg/minute). You then should order definitive diagnostic tests. In many institutions, this consists of an aortogram; others use MRI, contrast chest CT scanning, or transesophageal echocardiography. Patients with proximal dissection require surgery; those with distal dissection usually can be managed medically. If you suspect aortic dissection, immediately notify the cardiothoracic surgery team, or make arrangements for transfer.

Pulmonary Embolism

The pain of a PE is usually pleuritic but can be dull, mimicking a myocardial infarction (MI). These patients often complain of associated dyspnea. They may have hemoptysis. A history of immobility (e.g., a long plane flight), CHF, any underlying malignancy, or the use of cigarettes or birth control pills may be suggestive of PE. A personal or family history of deep venous thrombosis or a PE should raise your index of suspicion.

Physical examination may reveal tachypnea or tenderness and swelling in the legs. Less than half of patients with a PE are tachycardic, and their heart rates should not be used as a basis for diagnosis of PE. The ECG most commonly shows nonspecific ST-T changes or an $S_1Q_3T_3$ pattern. The chest x-ray may be normal, or it may show the classic "Hampton's hump" of pulmonary infarction (a wedge-shaped, pleural-based density) or Westermark's sign (increased central vascular markings with peripheral oligemia). An elevated hemidiaphragm may be seen. Blood gases usually show an increased A-a gradient and desaturation; however, 10% to 15% of patients may have totally normal blood gas values. **PEARL: Blood gas values never substitute for a V̇/Q̇ scan or a CT angiogram.**

The treatment for PE is IV heparinization, which should be started immediately if the diagnosis is strongly suspected, even before further diagnostic testing. An IV bolus of 80 U/kg followed by a continuous infusion of 18 U/kg per hour should be given and adjusted to achieve a partial thromboplastin time (PTT) 1.5 to 2 times the normal. Low-molecular-weight heparin (enoxaparin 1 mg/kg every 12 hours), given subcutaneously, is now also being used.

The diagnosis of PE can immediately be established in patients with a deep vein thrombosis by an abnormal lung $\dot{V}/\dot{Q}$ scan, an abnormal CT angiogram, or pulmonary angiography. The diagnosis of a PE is excluded in the patient who has a low clinical suspicion and a normal $\dot{V}/\dot{Q}$ scan. If the scan is abnormal in any way (i.e., with low or intermediate probability), the patient will need further tests to exclude a PE. Only the patient with high clinical suspicion and a high-probability scan should be treated for PE without further studies. Recently, there has been a trend toward use of Ëelical angiography. This modality identifies most PE as well as other diagnoses; however, it is less sensitive for peripheral PE.

Noninvasive studies of the legs looking for deep venous thrombosis also can be useful. In most cases, we start with lung scanning, followed by leg studies if the scan is nondiagnostic. If the leg studies are negative but we still strongly suspect PE, we then get a pulmonary angiogram. A proposed diagnostic approach to PE is presented in Figure 4–1.

Pneumothorax

Patients with pneumothorax can complain of sharp and pleuritic chest pain, often with associated dyspnea. Often, they are young, thin men. The lung examination may not show any abnormality, but the chest x-ray usually is diagnostic. It is sometimes helpful to get an end-expiratory film, which accentuates the abnormality. **PEARL: In children or uncooperative patients, a lateral decubitus film with the affected side up may also accentuate a pneumothorax.** Treatment usually involves placing a chest tube or a smaller "pigtail" catheter into the pleural space. **PEARL: If the pneumothorax is under tension, the patient is likely to be in serious trouble.**

After diagnosis, treatment should begin before you get the chest x-ray. Suspect tension pneumothorax in a patient with hypotension, tracheal deviation, jugular venous dis-

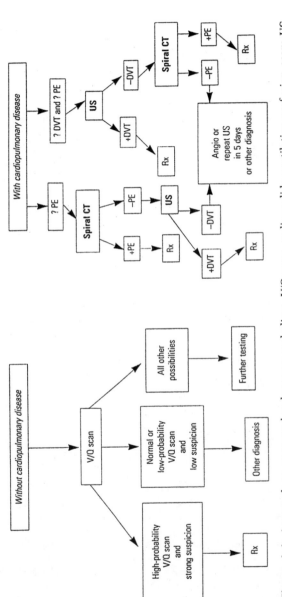

Figure 4-1. Approach to suspected pulmonary embolism. V/Q scan, radionuclide ventilation-perfusion scan; US, Doppler ultrasound; Rx, treatment; DVT, deep vein thrombosis; angio, pulmonary angiography; PE, pulmonary embolism. (From Holbert, Costello, & Federle: Spiral CT in the diagnosis of pulmonary embolism. *Ann Emergency Med* 1999, 33:526, with permission; as modified from Goodman, LR, et al: Acute pulmonary embolism: The role of computed tomographic imaging. *J Thorac Imag* 1997, 12:83–86.)

tention, and unilaterally decreased breath sounds. The treatment for pneumothorax is discussed in Chapter 3.

Esophageal Rupture

Patients with esophageal rupture usually complain of severe mid-chest pain following repeated bouts of vomiting. Physical examination generally is not helpful, but the patient may have a fever. Chest x-ray may show pneumo-mediastinum or a pleural effusion. The diagnosis of esophageal rupture must be made expeditiously; delay in diagnosis of more than 12 hours is associated with extremely high mortality because of the onset of mediastinitis. Early surgical consultation is mandatory. IV antibiotics should be given as soon as the diagnosis is established.

Myocardial Ischemia or Infarction

Myocardial ischemia and myocardial infarction are put together because, for the emergency physician, there is no difference in the disposition. Classically, these patients complain of dull or heavy substernal chest pain. Anginal pain usually is initiated by activity, whereas the pain of infarction generally begins when the patient is resting. Patients may have a history of cardiac disease or risk factors. Physical examination often is normal. Even the initial ECG may be normal or nonspecific in about 50% of patients with ischemia. Therefore, this diagnosis often hinges on history alone. **PEARL: A normal ECG and cardiac enzymes do not exclude cardiac disease.**

Treatment of angina involves the use of nitrates [nitroglycerin 0.4 mg sublingually (SL) every 5 minutes, or nitropaste 1 to 2 inches to chest wall, or IV nitroglycerin 10 to 200 µg/minute titrated to a 10% to 30% reduction in BP or pain relief] and aspirin (81 to 325 mg PO). Morphine 2 to 5 mg IV may be useful for pain that does not respond to nitrates. Our usual procedure is to treat the patient with a nitroglycerin tablet SL every 3 to 5 minutes to a total of three tablets; then if pain persists and the ECG is nondiagnostic, we treat the pain with morphine. In this case, you must repeat the ECG in about 30 minutes to see whether new and diagnostic changes have developed. Consider IV heparin or low-molecular-weight heparin in patients with ongoing pain or ECG evidence of ischemia. A glycoprotein IIb/IIIa inhibitor should also be considered with the cardiologist, especially if the patient is going for cardiac catheterization.

Treatment of an actual MI often requires thrombolytics [streptokinase 1,500,000 U IV, tissue plasminogen activator (t-PA) 100 mg IV or recombinant plasminogen factor (r-PA) 20 units, IV nitroglycerin, IV beta-blockers (metoprolol 5 mg IV every 5 minutes to a total of 15 mg), or cardiac catheterization with emergency angioplasty or coronary artery bypass]. Beta-blockers should be avoided in patients with cocaine-associated chest pain. Thrombolytic therapy is usually given if the ECG shows ST elevation of 1 mm or more in two or more contiguous leads and if the pain has lasted less than 12 hours. Before giving thrombolytics, be sure to ask the patient about contraindications, including active ulcer disease, surgery within the past 6 weeks, brain tumors or metastases, history of hemorrhagic stroke, bleeding disorders, or allergic reaction to thrombolytics, especially streptokinase. **PEARL: Look at the chest x-ray for mediastinal widening before giving thrombolytics.**

Patients with severe uncontrolled hypertension should have their BP controlled before thrombolytics are given. Even patients with ischemia who are not getting thrombolytics should receive aspirin or other platelet-inhibiting agents unless contraindicated.

DISPOSITION

Most patients with chest pain will be admitted to the hospital. You should only discharge patients who have a clear and nondangerous cause of their pain. **PEARL: Patients younger than 30 years with no drug use (e.g., cocaine) and with sharp, pleuritic, completely reproducible chest pain and a normal ECG are the only category of patients that you may safely discharge home nearly 100% of the time.** Despite emergency medicine's best efforts, approximately 5% of patients with MI are sent home inadvertently each year. If you practice with the mind-set that every chest pain is a potential MI and that each patient must prove to you that coronary artery disease is not responsible for this pain, you will minimize your miss rate. With MIs, you may not get a second chance to correct the mistake.

5

Shortness of Breath

PREHOSPITAL CONSIDERATIONS

▶ Field care is usually directed at treating bronchospasm or congestive heart failure (CHF).
▶ Other causes of shortness of breath (dyspnea) generally require further in-hospital workup and treatment, but EMS treatment for those two causes often markedly improves a patient's condition.
▶ In severe dyspnea or respiratory failure, paramedics usually need to intubate a patient in the field.
▶ Patients who are difficult to intubate may be ventilated with a bag-valve-mask.
▶ All patients with dyspnea should receive 100% supplemental oxygen.

As with chest pain, shortness of breath can reflect numerous diseases of varying severity. This chapter outlines some of the important aspects of working up the patient who is short of breath, but the discussion is not exhaustive by any means. The protocols that follow reflect our practice; workup and treatment may vary in other hospitals. A useful mnemonic for the causes of acute dyspnea is **PPOPPA:**

P pulmonary embolus (PE)
P pulmonary edema

O obstruction (e.g., foreign body, epiglottitis)
P pneumothorax
P pneumonia
A asthma or chronic obstructive pulmonary disease (COPD)

PEARL: Always consider pulmonary embolism in the differential diagnosis of dyspnea. Also, consider myocardial ischemia, even without chest pain, especially in the elderly.

PEARL: Consider foreign body aspiration in infants and children with dyspnea, especially if acute in onset.

HISTORY

For many of these conditions, the patient's history will give important clues. Patients with asthma usually are aware of their condition. A history of need for intubation or steroids in a patient with asthma suggests a more severe prognosis. Inquire about cough, fever, and other associated symptoms. Does the patient have orthopnea or paroxysmal nocturnal dyspnea? Is there a history of pedal edema? Ask about the risk factors for PE (see Chapter 4). Question the patient about exposure to tuberculosis and his or her purified protein derivative (PPD) status. Ask what medications the patient is taking. A long history of cigarette smoking suggests either COPD or lung cancer. **PEARL: Not all that wheezes is asthma and not all asthma wheezes.** All new "asthmatics" should be worked up for other causes.

PHYSICAL EXAMINATION

Physical examination for the patient with dyspnea can be very helpful. Fever usually is due to an infection but can appear with PE and many other disorders (e.g., MI, cancer). The lung examination is of course paramount, but don't neglect the cardiac examination, including looking for lateral displacement of the point of maximal impulse, jugular venous distention, and pedal edema, all of which suggest CHF. When examining the lungs, listen for rales, wheezes, bronchial breath sounds, decreased aeration, and egophony. Localized wheezes are suggestive of a bronchial foreign body. Percuss for dullness, and evaluate fremitus. Listen for stridor, because this is a very worrisome finding; it indicates some degree of upper airway obstruction. You should also beware of patients with "silent lungs" who do not have wheezes or rales; this may reflect limited air movement.

ANCILLARY TESTS

For patients with a history of asthma or COPD, bedside measurement of peak flow can be useful, especially if the patient's usual values are known. Pulse oximetry is a quick, cheap, and noninvasive way to evaluate lung function. Measure O_2 saturation for every patient with dyspnea. Be aware, though, that the reading tells you only about oxygenation and not ventilation (for which you need the CO_2 tension from a blood gas). Also, patients can have a "normal" saturation (e.g., 94%) and still have low blood O_2 tension (in this example, the Po_2 may be in the 60s, and therefore a major A-a gradient may be present. In any patient who has an abnormal pulse oximeter reading (below about 95%) or in whom you suspect moderate to severe lung disease, consider an ABG.

The most important other diagnostic test for the patient with dyspnea is the chest x-ray. In patients with chronic lung disease, try to get old films for comparison. Other tests to consider include an ECG, if cardiac disease is suspected, or the PE workup (see Chapter 4 for more details).

DIFFERENTIAL DIAGNOSIS

One diagnostic dilemma you may face in the older dyspneic patient is differentiating between CHF and COPD. Both conditions can produce wheezing, but the therapies are markedly different. **PEARL: History and medication use may help differentiate COPD and CHF.** A chest x-ray often is extremely helpful. In patients whose film shows mild CHF but whose examination is more consistent with COPD, consider a trial of bronchodilators. An ECG should be obtained in such patients prior to giving beta-agonists to exclude cardiac ischemia. Obtain old records to help sort things out. If you are still unsure and the patient is hemodynamically stable, you can try giving nitroglycerin SL to reduce preload. This will help in CHF, but not in COPD.

TREATMENT

Asthma

Measure respiratory rate, heart rate, and peak flow, and assess the patient's color and use of accessory muscles. Use these variables to monitor the patient's response to therapy after each intervention. Begin treatment with nebulized beta-agonists. We use albuterol 2.5 mg in adults and children older than 5 years (1.25 to 2.5 in younger children), repeated every 10 to 20 minutes as long as no cardiovascular problems ensue. Nebulized ipratropium bromide may have synergistic effects and should be added in all patients. Steroids should be given early to all patients who are currently on steroids or have used them recently, patients with severe asthma, and in most patients with prolonged symptoms.

If there has been a steady improvement in the patient's condition and the peak flow is greater than 70% of predicted value for age and size, discharge the patient on a short course of oral steroids, such as prednisone 40 to 60 mg/day for 5 days (adult). Often, no tapering is required. Although use of a metered-dose inhaler in older children and adults is appropriate, use of a spacer improves drug delivery and should be considered, especially in young children.

If peak flow remains below 40% of predicted, give IV corticosteroids (e.g., methylprednisolone 2 mg/kg up to 125 mg) and admit the patient to the hospital. Patients with severe asthma and increasing CO_2 levels may need to be intubated. Intubation can sometimes be avoided in severe cases if you administer beta-agonists systemically [epinephrine 0.3 mg subcutaneously (SC)] or IV magnesium sulfate 2 g over 20 to 30 minutes. If intubation is required, induction with ketamine is appropriate (see Chapter 2).

For patients with intermediate peak flow values, therapy can involve discharge on oral steroids, but keep a low threshold for admitting any of these patients. Any patient with active asthma and a concurrent lung disease, such as pneumonia, should be admitted.

Anaphylaxis

Patients with anaphylaxis usually have a history of allergy to some substance known to them to trigger these attacks, such as bee stings or foods such as peanuts. They can present with severe facial swelling, stridor, wheezing, and hypotension. If treated rapidly, they can recover quickly. If the patient at any point requires intubation or develops hypotension, ICU admission is mandatory. The most common cause of true anaphylaxis is still penicillin.

A usual course is to begin therapy for early anaphylaxis with epinephrine 1:1,000 solution 0.3 to 0.5 mL SC (0.01 mg/kg SC in children). Follow this with 50 mg IV diphenhydramine (1.0 mg/kg in children). Patients with wheezing can benefit from nebulized beta-agonists. Be cautious with epinephrine in any patient with suspected coronary artery disease, but remember that anaphylaxis can kill, so be prepared to use epinephrine.

Any patient who has no history of hypotension and no dyspnea or stridor following treatment may be given one dose of IV corticosteroids. In addition, the patient may be discharged on oral corticosteroids (such as prednisone as outlined previously for asthma in adults) and diphenhydramine (often 25 to 50 mg every 6 hours for adults) for several days. Observe such patients for about 4 to 6 hours before discharge to ensure that they do not relapse before the steroids begin to take effect. All other patients should receive IV corticosteroids and be admitted. An H_2-blocker, such as cimetidine 300 mg IV, may have additional benefit.

Hypotensive patients require epinephrine 1:10,000 solution 1 to 10 mL slow IV push to reverse life-threatening shock. They also require fluids, such as up to 6 liters of Ringer's lactate can be required.

Pulmonary Edema

The treatment modalities for pulmonary edema can be summarized by the mnemonic **LMNOP:**

L   Lasix (furosemide) IV one or two times the patient's usual dose, or 40 mg if the patient is not usually on the drug.

M   morphine, given in doses of 2 to 4 mg IV. Avoid respiratory depression.

N   nitroglycerin, often given IV; may be given sublingually every 2 minutes while the drip is being prepared. Start with 5 to 10 μg/minute IV and increase by 5 μg/minute every 3 to 5 minutes. Hypotension should be avoided.

O oxygen; 100% O_2 should be given to all patients with pulmonary edema.

P position. The patient should be, and will want to be, sitting up.

In general, start therapy with the patient in an upright position with O_2, nitroglycerin SL, and IV furosemide. If the patient does not improve, start IV nitroglycerin at a rate of 10 μg/min, titrating to a 10% to 30% decrease in the mean arterial pressure. Give small doses of morphine to anxious patients. Throughout the treatment, follow the patient's pulmonary status (e.g., by pulse oximeter), RR, and urine output (which may require bladder catheterization). Get ABG values, ECG, and chest x-ray early.

Consider intubation if the patient is worsening clinically, has deteriorating mental status, or remains hypoxic, acidotic, or hypercarbic despite aggressive therapy. **PEARL: Before intubating, consider noninvasive positive-pressure ventilation methods. BIPAP (bilevel positive airway pressure) or CPAP (continuous positive airway pressure) masks are effective treatments, which may prevent intubation.** Most patients with PE are admitted to the ICU. Some may go to a monitored stepdown unit, a few may be able to go to an unmonitored bed, and only stable, chronic patients are discharged home.

6
CHAPTER

Abdominal Pain

PREHOSPITAL CONSIDERATIONS

▶ Abdominal pain is a common cause for patients to call EMS. Patients with the most catastrophic illnesses need hospital or operative resources.

▶ It is best not to use analgesia in the field until the patient has been appropriately evaluated in the ED.

▶ Beware of the patient complaining of abdominal pain who may be having an acute MI or a ruptured abdominal aortic aneurysm. Monitor the patient's vital signs carefully and rapidly transport to the ED.

Abdominal pain is a very challenging symptom to work up in the ED because of the broad differential diagnoses. This chapter does not include a detailed discussion of the many entities that can cause abdominal pain; instead, it focuses on some of the more pertinent points in the workup. Most important is that you do not miss serious disease, even if you cannot specifically diagnose the problem immediately. **PEARL: When evaluating a patient, always consider life-threatening conditions.** Be aware that the usual presenting signs and symptoms may be altered or absent in children, the elderly, AIDS patients, the mentally handicapped, and any patient on corticosteroid therapy or with a chronic condition. It is best to be conservative with these patients, and in all those in whom a specific diagnosis cannot be established. **PEARL: Elderly patients may not exhibit classic signs**

and symptoms of serious abdominal disorders; therefore, always have a high index of suspicion for serious disorders.

HISTORY

The history is crucial to the diagnosis. Ask about the time course, character, and location of the pain, including whether it has changed in any of these variables over time. The time and severity of the onset may help distinguish vascular or catastrophic conditions. Vascular or visceral ruptures occur abruptly; other pains start more gradually. Associated symptoms (e.g., nausea, anorexia, fever, diarrhea, vomiting, vaginal bleeding or discharge, and dysuria) may be important. Inquire as to how food affects the pain. Most people inappropriately associate any abdominal problem with whatever they ate last. Find out when the patient last ate; this will be important if surgery is necessary. Note any alcohol intake or medications (e.g., NSAIDs), which can cause abdominal irritation or disorders. Change in bowel habits with significant weight loss may suggest an intra-abdominal malignancy. Ask about previous surgery, anatomic abnormalities, or a history of aortic aneurysm. Always ask any woman when her last menstrual period began and whether it was normal for her or irregular or unusual in some way. **PEARL: All women of childbearing age are pregnant and those with abdominal pain have an ectopic pregnancy until proven otherwise.**

PHYSICAL EXAMINATION

The physical examination should establish whether the patient has "an acute surgical abdomen" (i.e., peritoneal signs such as rebound, rigidity, or guarding). Evaluate the patient's general appearance. Is the patient moaning in pain, or chewing on cheese doodles? Is the patient diaphoretic, pale, or ashen? Doubled over or moving about the bed trying to find a comfortable position? When examining for rebound, be as gentle as possible. It is sometimes helpful to percuss other than at the site of tenderness to see if that causes an increase in discomfort. For all patients, the examination must include a rectal and genitourinary examination; a pelvic examination also must be performed in female patients. Vital signs are important to note—any fever, hypotension, tachycardia, or increased respiratory rate. Palpation may be the only means to help with a diagnosis. Palpation should be gentle, examining for involuntary guarding. In patients who are ticklish, placing the examining hand over the patient's hand during examination may significantly reduce the likelihood of tickling the patient. It is important to distract the patient and examine the "tender" area many times to check for consistency. Check for masses and organomegaly. Specific signs may also be helpful, but simple tenderness in the right upper quadrant (RUQ) or right lower quadrant (RLQ) does not make a diagnosis. Midinspiratory apnea on deep palpation of the RUQ suggests an inflamed gallbladder. Rovsing's sign is pain in the RLQ while palpating the left lower abdomen; it can be present in a patient with acute appendicitis. When palpating for a pulsatile mass of the aorta, use two hands, with the fingertips pressing directly on top of the aorta. Feel the pulses push the fingertips up and down. Then move the hands gradually apart until you feel the pulsation pushing your hands apart. You should be able to determine whether the width of the aorta is more than 6 cm. Also, remember to do a complete chest examination; more than one person has been fooled by a lower lobe pneumonia presenting as upper abdominal pain. Always percuss for tenderness at the costovertebral angles.

ANCILLARY TESTS

Lab work in general may be helpful but is rarely diagnostic. It should include a CBC, electrolytes, glucose, blood urea nitrogen (BUN) and creatinine, amylase or lipase, liver enzymes (possibly), and a urinalysis. The absence of a leukocytosis does not rule out an intra-abdominal infection such as appendicitis. All women of childbearing age must have a pregnancy test, even if they tell you they couldn't possibly be pregnant. Order a chest x-ray for older patients and young children who have abdominal pain. An upright chest x-ray is the appropriate study to exclude free intra-abdominal gas; if the patient cannot sit or stand, get a left-lateral abdominal decubitus film for this purpose (air will be outlined against the liver). Abdominal films are rarely useful unless you suspect obstruction, but occasionally, they can be helpful in cases of renal and biliary tract disease, in which you would be looking for abnormal calcifications. Further studies such as IV pyelography, ultrasonography, and abdominal CT scanning are very diagnosis- and institution-dependent. Ultrasound can be useful for determining gallbladder disease or renal hydronephrosis. It is also very useful for discovering the cause of pelvic pain in women. Noncontrast CT is a fast, noninvasive means of quickly verifying the presence of urinary calculi.

DIFFERENTIAL DIAGNOSIS

The location of pain may help focus the differential diagnosis. Table 6–1 lists some diagnostic considerations for the differential diagnosis.

Cholecystitis

Acute cholecystitis is almost always (95%) due to gallstones. Acalculous cholecystitis is typically found only in

Table 6–1. DIFFERENTIAL DIAGNOSIS OF ABDOMINAL PAIN

Location	Possible Diagnoses
Right upper quadrant (RUQ)	Hepatitis, cholecystitis or biliary colic, pancreatitis, perforated ulcer, right lower lobar pneumonia, myocardial infarction (MI)
Left upper quadrant (LUQ)	Peptic ulcer; gastritis; pancreatitis; splenic enlargement; rupture or infarction; left lower lobar pneumonia, MI
Midepigastric	Ulcer, pancreatitis, dyspeptic syndromes, MI
Right lower quadrant (RLQ)	Appendicitis, cecal volvulus, strangulated inguinal hernia, mesenteric adenitis, ectopic pregnancy, gynecologic pathology, testicular torsion
Left lower quadrant (LLQ)	Diverticulitis, colitis (infectious or inflammatory), gynecologic pathology, testicular torsion
Anywhere	Ischemic bowel, inflammatory bowel disease, diabetic ketoacidosis, gastroenteritis

elderly or debilitated patients. Pain is often of sudden on-set and radiating from the RUQ to the back or the scapula. The condition usually is associated with anorexia, nausea, and vomiting. The patient's RUQ is tender. Fever often is present after 1 to 2 days of pain, but rarely before. Similar pain lasting only a few hours is usually due to biliary colic (i.e., gallstone impaction and then passage), a precursor to acute cholecystitis. An inspiratory arrest on deep palpation below the right costal margin (Murphy's sign) is commonly found. Patients may, however, present without any fever or leukocytosis.

Ultrasound can demonstrate the presence of gallstones, but it is only 80% to 90% sensitive for acute cholecystitis (evidenced by gallbladder wall thickening and the presence of pericholecystic fluid). The test of choice to exclude acute cholecystitis is hepatoiminodiacetic acid (HIDA) scanning. This test is positive when the isotope is unable to enter the cystic duct to fill the gallbladder; if the gallbladder is visualized, acute cholecystitis is excluded.

Patients with acute cholecystitis require hospital admission for IV antibiotics and surgery. Patients with pain typical of biliary colic, but without acute cholecystitis and whose pain resolves, may be discharged with a surgical follow-up arranged.

Hepatitis

Hepatitis can have a subacute course of days to weeks. It can be caused by either toxic exposures (e.g., ethanol, ac-etaminophen) or viral infection. The patient may have jaundice, RUQ pain, anorexia, nausea, and/or a low-grade fever. Liver enzymes are elevated. Liver function should be assessed by checking coagulation parameters (PT and PTT).

Patients with hepatitis may not require admission in all cases, but they do require at least close follow-up with an internist or gastroenterologist. Admission is indicated in the following circumstances:

- Fulminant hepatitis with encephalopathy
- Severe vomiting and diarrhea with severe dehydration requiring IV hydration
- PT prolonged > 3 seconds above normal
- Hypoglycemia
- Bilirubin >20 mg/dL

- The elderly patient
- Immunosuppression
- Uncertain diagnosis

Watch for the alcoholic patient with RUQ pain. These patients may have a low-grade fever, jaundice, and tender hepatomegaly. A thorough search for other infectious diseases, such as pneumonia, urinary tract infection, sepÛis, meningitis, and subacute bacterial peritonitis (SBP) is required. Any such patient with an altered mental status, fever, encephalopathy, or increasing abdominal girth requires a peritoneal tap and evaluation for SBP.

Peptic Ulcer Disease

Patients with peptic ulcer disease or gastritis may present with epigastric or LUQ pain, sometimes radiating to the back. Cigarettes and alcohol use is strongly associated with these disorders. The pain is often relieved with antacids. Exclude active or severe bleeding (by checking for rectal occult blood, nasogastric aspirate, orthostatic vital signs, and hematocrit) and perforation (either by examination or by chest x-ray for free air).

Many patients with inferior wall MIs present with symptoms similar to those of peptic ulcer disease. All patients, especially those with cardiac risk factors, must receive an ECG to check for cardiac ischemia.

If all of the latter problems are excluded, the patient may be discharged on antacids (to be given 1 and 3 hours after meals and before bedtime) and H_2-blockers (cimetidine 400 to 800 mg every night or ranitidine 150 mg twice daily) with close follow-up.

Pancreatitis

Pancreatitis most often is caused by alcohol, gallstone impaction, trauma, or drug toxicity (e.g., thiazide diuretics, pentamidine, corticosteroids, and zidovudine). Patients present with severe epigastric pain radiating to the back and often nausea and vomiting. The epigastric area is usually tender, and rebound tenderness and guarding may be present. In severe cases, the patient may be in shock. Serum amylase and/or lipase is often elevated.

Most patients with pancreatitis should be admitted and

receive IV fluid hydration and pain management. The use of a nasogastric tube to prevent vomiting and to rest the bowel is controversial. Additional laboratory tests that are helpful in determining the patient's prognosis include WBC count, lactic dehydrogenase (LDH), aspartate transaminase (AST), calcium, and glucose.

Appendicitis

Appendicitis classically presents as crampy periumbilical pain, which, over a period of 12 to 24 hours, localizes to the RLQ and becomes steady and sharp as peritoneal irritation occurs.

Affected patients often have anorexia and a low-grade fever. **PEARL: The classic presentation of appendicitis is rare in the very young, the very old, and pregnant women.** Always maintain a high index of suspicion for this disease in any patient with abdominal pain, and observe them for several hours with repeated examinations if you are not sure. No tests are sensitive enough to be useful in diagnosing appendicitis. Many studies suggest that anorexia is present in all cases of appendicitis and that the WBC count is usually elevated. These findings may be helpful when they are present, but not finding them does not exclude the diagnosis. Therefore, appendicitis still remains a clinical diagnosis; with minimal suspicion, obtain a surgical consultation. In experienced hands, RLQ ultrasonography can be very helpful in questionable cases; however, contrast CT of the abdomen has been shown to be more useful in making the diagnosis of appendicitis. Patients with obvious peritoneal signs should be taken to the operating room without major delays.

Diverticulitis

Diverticulitis often is called "left-sided appendicitis," and patients present with symptoms very similar to those associated with acute appendicitis, although diverticulitis is more commonly associated with LLQ findings. Similar cautions apply. Generally, consider diverticulitis in elderly patients with abdominal pain and fever. Patients should be admitted if they have complicated diverticulitis, in which surgical intervention is necessary for abscesses, perforations, fistulas, and obstructions.

Ischemic Bowel Disease

Ischemic bowel is also more common in elderly patients, who often have atherosclerotic disease, and in patients who are predisposed to thrombosis. It typically presents as pain out of proportion with physical findings. Although abdominal x-ray may (rarely) show "thumb-printing" of the bowel wall, this diagnosis is hard to establish because most of the lab findings are nonspecific (elevated WBC or amylase) or late (acidosis). In elderly patients with abdominal pain, maintain a high index of suspicion for ischemic bowel disease, and pursue it aggressively by ruling out other diseases and getting an early surgical consultation. Although abdominal CT may be helpful, angiography may be required for a definitive diagnosis. **PEARL: Beware of the elderly patient with atrial fibrillation, in whom emboli may be thrown to the mesenteric arteries.**

Gastroenteritis

Gastroenteritis is a common discharge diagnosis for patients with abdominal pain for whom no cause was determined. Be aware that the cardinal symptoms of this disease—most often due to a viral infection—are vomiting and diarrhea. Without these symptoms, it usually is better to discharge the patient with the diagnosis of "abdominal pain of unknown cause" rather than give all concerned the false security of an erroneous diagnosis. All such patients should be closely followed up. Many disorders can cause nausea and vomiting (from glaucoma to intestinal obstructions), so it is essential that you fully evaluate these patients. **PEARL: Beware of the diagnosis of "gastroenteritis." It is usually a diagnosis of exclusion and may represent an underlying catastrophic illness.**

Abdominal Aortic aneurysm

Abdominal aortic aneurysms (AAA) are most commonly seen in elderly patients with hypertension or atherosclerotic disease. **PEARL: Ruptured AAAs have a high mortality, and early diagnosis with rapid surgical intervention is necessary.** Although they are often asymptomatic, AAAs may manifest as abdominal, back, or testicular pain, especially when they are leaking or have ruptured. Patients with a leaking AAA classically present with abdominal pain, hypotension, and a pulsatile mass. Hemodynamically unstable patients with suspected AAA should be taken to the OR without further delay. In stable patients, an abdominal CT should be obtained. When rapidly available, a bedside US can help expedite workup and management. All patients with a suspected ruptured AAA should have emergency surgical consultation, and intravenous access should be rapidly established.

MANAGEMENT AND DISPOSITION

All patients with an "acute abdomen" (i.e., rebound, guarding, and rigidity) should have an immediate surgical consultation. Other patients with abdominal pain should have a period of observation in the ED unless a clear nonsurgical cause of the pain is found or the pain resolves over the course of the ED visit. ED observational units have allowed greater workups and extended observation for patients with abdominal pain as an alternative to hospital admission. If the pain persists, an early surgical consultation can help expedite the disposition of many patients with abdominal pain. It is better to involve the surgeon earlier rather than later. Many surgeons prefer that patients do not receive pain medication before their examination, although some data show that medication actually improves the examination (by making the patient more comfortable and cooperative). This is a matter best discussed with your consultants to see what they prefer. If the diagnosis is unclear and the patient continues to have abdominal pain, consider hospital admission for further diagnostic workup. **PEARL: Up to half of the patients in the ED will not have a clear diagnosis, and extended observation or admission may be prudent.**

Unless a clear and benign diagnosis is made, it is safe to discharge patients with abdominal pain only if they appear well, can tolerate oral fluids, and can be reliably observed at home by a companion (who would be able to summon help if necessary). For these patients, detailed warnings and instructions should be given, and follow-up within 24 hours should be arranged. Patients discharged from the ED with nonspecific abdominal pain must be given instructions to return to the ED if their symptoms worsen and do not improve.

7
CHAPTER

Neurologic Problems

PREHOSPITAL CONSIDERATIONS

▶ Patients with neurologic problems require rapid transfer with support of vital functions.
▶ Assess ABCs, with particular emphasis on a patient's ability to support his or her airway. For patients with an altered mental status, determine a rapid bedside glucose. If unavailable, give 50-mL intravenous bolus of 50% dextrose along with naloxone (Narcan) 2 mg IV and thiamine 100 mg IV.
▶ Patients with a history of seizures who have a single noncomplex seizure and short postictal state typical of their seizure do not need to be transported to the hospital.
▶ Patients with any atypical or multiple seizures need to be transported and evaluated in the ED.

COMA

The initial approach to an unconscious patient differs from the traditional clinical assessment technique. Even *before* all the information about a patient is known, one may have to:

1. Stabilize basic life functions (ABCs).
2. Protect the patient from further harm.
3. Promptly treat reversible disorders.

PEARL: Obtain an early bedside glucose on all patients with altered mental status or focal neurologic deficits.

The initial phase of resuscitation should follow the ABC format. Ensure that the patient has an open airway and is breathing; this may require intubation. Assess oxygenation by pulse oximetry, and give supplemental oxygen as necessary. Look for and treat hypotension, if necessary. Obtain IV access and draw blood for the lab. Do an immediate chemstrip test for glucose, if available. Give 2 mg of naloxone and 100 mg of thiamine IV. If the bedside glucose reading was low or if you cannot perform that test, give 50 mL of 50% dextrose in water ($D_{50}W$) IV (in children 4 mL/kg of $D_{25}W$ IV). At this point, assuming that you have successfully treated the abnormalities noted during your primary survey, you can go on to a more detailed evaluation.

History and Physical Examination

- Whatever history can be obtained is vital. Question the people who found or brought in the patient about the circumstances in which he or she was found. **PEARL: Get history from acquaintances of all comatose patients.**
- Were any convulsions noted?
- Is there a history of seizures?
- Did the patient complain of anything before collapsing?
- Were any drugs, toxins, or alcohol found nearby or known to be available?
- What medical history is known?
- What is the patient's baseline mental status?
- Was there a rapid or progressive change in mental status?
- Is there any deterioration since they first saw the patient?
- Was there any evidence of trauma?

Do a general physical examination, looking especially for fever or rashes (consider meningococcemia or meningitis), needle marks (IV drug use), oral burns (toxic ingestion), nuchal rigidity, and signs of trauma (e.g., hemotympanum). Perform a rectal exam to look for occult blood. The neurologic exam should assess the following:

- **Respiratory pattern:** Apneustic or ataxic breathing indicates a brain-stem injury, whereas Cheyne-Stokes breathing indicates bilateral hemispheric disease.
- **Pupillary reactivity:** Check pupil size, symmetry, and reactivity to light.

- **Extraocular movements:** Also perform the cold-caloric test. Look into the ears to exclude tympanic membrane perforation; then instill 15 to 30 mL of ice water into each ear canal while watching the eyes. The normal brain stem drives the eyes slowly toward this stimulus, and the normal hemispheres then cause nystagmus away from the stimulus. Hence, a patient with bilateral hemispheric injury or disease, as in poisoning or hypoxia, will show only a slow movement toward the ice water. The unresponsive patient who has suffered structural damage to the brain stem will have no response to cold stimulation (Fig. 7–1). **PEARL: Obtain an imaging study on all patients with lateralizing signs.**
- **Motor tone:** Look especially for asymmetry of tone, which indicates a localized structural lesion. Look also for decorticate or decerebrate posturing (Fig. 7–2).

Calculate a GCS score (see Chapter 3) on every patient. If the patient has to be sedated, paralyzed, or intubated, try to assess these variables very quickly before that intervention. Just say to the patient, "Open your eyes! What's your name?" Observe the response to supraorbital pressure or other noxious stimuli (one that works very well is the insertion of a cotton swab into the posterior nasopharynx). The GCS has some prognostic use for a patient who may require neurosurgical intervention.

The mnemonic **AEIOUTIPS** helps you remember the various causes of coma:

A alcohols and ingested drugs and toxins
E endocrine abnormalities, electrolyte disorders, and epilepsy
I intoxication, insulin deficiency (diabetes)
O oxygen deficiency and opioids
U uremia
T trauma, tumor
I infection
P psychiatric and porphyria
S stroke, shock, and subarachnoid hemorrhage

Ancillary Tests

Lab tests should include CBC, chemistries (including calcium and magnesium), ABGs, ECG, and CT scan of the

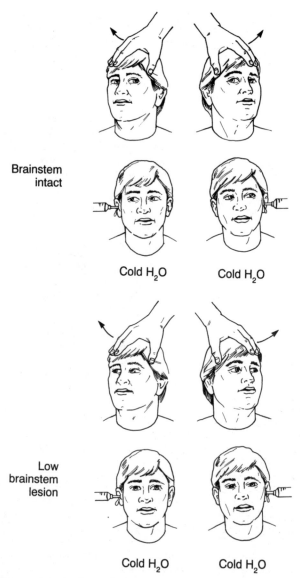

Brainstem
intact

Cold H$_2$O   Cold H$_2$O

Low
brainstem
lesion

Cold H$_2$O   Cold H$_2$O

Figure 7–1. Ocular reflexes and caloric testing in the unconscious patient.

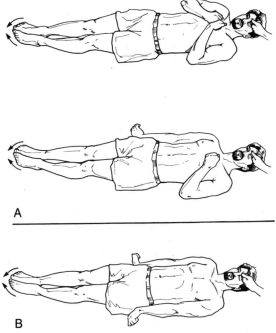

Figure 7–2. Decorticate (A) and decerebrate (B) posturing in response to a painful stimulus.

head. If meningitis is suspected, a lumbar puncture (LP) should be performed. Timing of the LP is sometimes controversial because there is a theoretic risk of herniation if the ICP is elevated. Studies have shown that it is safe to perform an LP before a CT without clinical evidence of increased ICP. Some prefer to wait for the CT scan. If you choose to wait, but you think meningitis is a real possibility, draw blood cultures and give antibiotics immediately! You can then do the LP within 2 hours and at least get a sample for a Gram's stain and immunoelectrophoresis of bacterial antigens. Other cerebrospinal fluid tests to send include the cell count (looking for infection or hemorrhage), glucose (low in infection), and protein (elevated in infection or some neurologic diseases), and culture. Toxicologic screens and an ethanol level should be considered, as indicated by the particular circumstances and findings.

Disposition

Comatose patients should be admitted to an ICU, or to the operating room if a neurosurgical emergency is found on the head CT scan. In very rare cases, when a treatable cause is found and the patient recovers rapidly, admission to a floor bed or discharge is possible.

SEIZURES

Patients who have a history of seizures and who have seized need no specific workup, other than a drug level when appropriate, with adjustment of medication doses when necessary. This section briefly outlines our approach to the actively "seizing" patient without head trauma. Each step, unless otherwise noted, assumes that the seizures are still continuing. Throughout the care of the patient, we assume that you will constantly be reassessing the patient's ABCs. Remember to test anticonvulsant levels if the patient has been receiving such therapy, as the most common reason for a seizure is inadequate blood levels of a prescribed anticonvulsant. Pertinent lab tests in patients with a first-time seizure should include CBC; electrolytes; calcium, magnesium, and glucose levels; BUN and creatinine levels; and CT scan of the head. The treatment protocol for seizures is as follows:

1. Evaluate the ABCs. Look for and treat hypoxia, hypotension, and hypoglycemia.
2. Establish IV access, and give thiamine 100 mg IV.
3. Give lorazepam 0.05 mg/kg (usually 4 mg in an adult) IV over 2 minutes.
4. In 3 to 5 minutes, repeat the same dose of lorazepam if the seizure is continuing.
5. Give phenytoin 15 to 18 mg/kg (usually 1 g in an adult) IV slowly, no *faster* than 0.5 mg/kg per minute. Monitor very closely for hypotension; if it occurs, stop the drip until it resolves; then resume at a slower rate. The same dosage of fosphenytoin can be given at a rate of 100 to 150 mg/kg per minute with fewer side effects.
6. If the seizure continues, give phenobarbital, 15 to 18 mg/kg IV, at 1 mg/kg per minute. This may be repeated to a maximum 30 mg/kg, if necessary.
7. By this point, neurologic consultation should be available. If seizures continue, consider clonazepam, paraldehyde, barbiturate coma, lidocaine, a midazolam drip, or

general anesthesia with electroencephalographic (EEG) monitoring.

STROKE

Think of stroke as a "brain attack" in which time is critical for maximal brain salvage, similar to the situation with MI. A patient who has had a cerebrovascular event usually presents with a focal neurologic deficit, such as aphasia or hemiparesis. Your first priority, as always, is to stabilize the patient (i.e., the ABCs). Some patients require intubation for altered mental status; all patients with possible stroke should receive oxygen. Ensure that the patient is hemodynamically stable. Begin cardiac monitoring. Look for and treat hypoglycemia. Obtain IV access and order an ECG because occasionally an MI can present as an embolic stroke from a ventricular thrombus. After the patient is stabilized, a further diagnostic workup can be carried out. **PEARL: Immediate noncontrast CT scanning of the head is mandatory to rule out a hemorrhage.**

In general, there are three types of strokes:

- *Hemorrhagic stroke* patients generally present with severe headache; such patients often are hypertensive.`Vomiting and nuchal rigidity may be present. A preceding headache can be noted.
- *Thrombotic stroke* is seen in patients with severe carotid atherosclerosis; they often present with a history of several hours or days of progressing symptoms.
- *Embolic stroke*, the most common, usually occurs in inadequately anticoagulated patients who have atrial fibrillation, a recent MI with a mural thrombus, or cardiac ventricular aneurysms. They can experience sudden onset of an unchanging symptom complex. All patients with stroke should be admitted for monitoring and treatment.

A *transient ischemic attack* (TIA) is a stroke-like syndrome that lasts less than 24 hours. A *reversible ischemic neurologic deficit* (RIND) lasts more than 24 hours but clears completely. Obviously, these diagnoses may be made only in retrospect. In general, a patient who presents with a resolving or resolved neurologic deficit that is stroke-like should be treated the same as a patient with a persistent deficit.

Treatment of ischemic strokes within 3 hours of onset with thrombolytics (t-PA 0.9 mg/kg up to 90 mg IV, 10% as a bolus with the remainder given as a drip over 60 minutes) improves clinical outcome. Performance of a CT to exclude intracranial hemorrhage is mandatory before giving t-PA. Anticoagulation and antiplatelet drugs should be withheld for 24 hours after t-PA. Contraindications to t-PA include recent head trauma or major surgery, history of intracranial bleeding, recent GI bleeding, uncontrolled hypertension (systolic pressure >185, diastolic pressure >110), and associated seizure.

NONTRAUMATIC HEADACHE

Patients who present to the ED with headache want pain relief. They also may be worried that they have a brain tumor, and they may want a CT scan or MRI of their brain. In general, most of them do not need any studies, but certain H&P findings should prompt you to pursue the possibility of serious disease aggressively.

Patients with headache and fever should be assessed extremely carefully for meningitis. Ask about photophobia or vomiting. Look for meningismus. If you suspect meningitis, an LP is mandatory, unless the patient has signs of increased ICP (e.g., papilledema) or focal neurologic deficits. In those cases, draw blood cultures, give antibiotics, and order a CT scan of the head to rule out a mass lesion before performing the LP. The presence of lateralizing signs or papilledema require imaging before LP.

Any headache patient with new focal neurologic deficits or confusion or with a severe sudden-onset headache should have a CT scan of the head. Look for subarachnoid hemorrhage. **PEARL: Perform lumbar puncture in patients with significant headaches yet normal imaging studies.** Immunosuppressed patients and those with a history consistent with tumor (a prolonged course of slowly worsening headache, especially on awakening) also should have a head CT, as should any patient with chronic headache who has a new type of headache (unless an obviously benign cause is found). **PEARL: Obtain an imaging study for worst-ever and sudden-onset headaches.**

Migraine

Migraine is a very common reason for patients with headache to present to the ED. Often, the pain is typical of their migraine headaches but worse in intensity and unresponsive to their available home therapies.

Migraine headaches are hemicranial and throbbing, and can be associated with photophobia, phonophobia, nausea, and vomiting. Many treatment options are available. Finding out what has helped the patient during previous visits to the ED can give you a good idea of what treatment to give. Many other options are available as well.

We like to use prochlorperazine (Compazine) 5 to 10 mg IV (in an adult) as a first-line agent, especially for those with nausea accompanying the headache; if that hasn't improved the pain in 20 minutes, we give dihydroergotamine (DHE) 1 mg IV. This drug is a vasoconstrictor and cannot be given to patients with coronary or cerebrovascular disease. Another option is sumatriptan 6 mg SC; this may be repeated once if the first dose doesn't work. Note that sumatriptan is also a vasoconstrictor with the same cautions as DHE. Various oral or intranasal formulations of DHE and sumatriptan are now available, too. Finally, of course, one can use IM or IV analgesics such as morphine; this usually relieves pain primarily by putting the patient to sleep. Before treating these patients with an opioid analgesic, which may mask subtle neurologic findings, these patients must have a complete history and neurologic examination.

8

CHAPTER

Acute Eye Problems

PREHOSPITAL CONSIDERATIONS

▸ Patients with penetrating injuries to the eye should have their eye covered with a firm shield.
▸ Copious eye irrigation in all chemical exposures should be performed at the scene in all stable patients.

PEARL: If a patient has any eye complaints, always check his or her visual acuity before examining the rest of the eye, except with obvious severe trauma such as a pencil penetrating the eyeball. Always assess pupillary response and extraocular movements, and look for foreign bodies under both upper and lower lids. The upper eyelid should always be everted over a cotton swab to exclude foreign bodies. Slit-lamp examination (Fig. 8–1) and fluorescein staining, direct ophthalmoscopy, and ocular pressure measurement complete the eye examination. Topical anesthesia, such as tetracaine or proparacaine eye drops, may assist you in performing the examination. In some cases, progressive swelling of the eyelids may make examination of the eyes difficult. **PEARL: Examine eyes early before swelling increases. Use retractors to open eyes that are swollen shut.** Also, consider and look for systemic disorders such as temporal arteritis in the patient with eye pain.

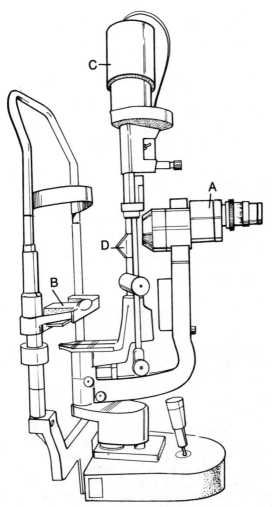

Figure 8–1. The slit lamp: (A) stereoscopic microscope; (B) patient's chin rest; (C) light source; (D) adjustable slit mechanism.

True ophthalmologic emergencies that always require immediate consultation include:

- Acute visual loss
- Chemical burns to the eye
- Penetrating eye injuries
- Acute angle closure glaucoma

THE RED EYE

Most patients with a red eye have a relatively benign cause (e.g., conjunctivitis). Patients with serious diseases may present with predominantly nonocular complaints. **PEARL: Look for red eyes in patients with headache, abdominal pain, or vomiting of unknown cause to exclude glaucoma.** The diagnosis of a red eye may be sorted out based on whether vision is affected.

Vision Decreased

Narrow-Angle Glaucoma

This is a true emergency. Patients with narrow-angle glaucoma have extremely high intraocular pressure (>20 mm Hg). They also have decreased vision, photophobia, eye pain, nausea, and vomiting. They often complain of seeing halos around lights. The pupil is fixed, and the cornea is often cloudy or "steamy." **PEARL: Think of glaucoma when the cornea is cloudy.** Obtain an immediate ophthalmologic consultation. Begin treatment with pilocarpine eye drops, beta-blocker eye drops, IV acetazolamide (500 mg), and IV mannitol (1 g/kg).

Uveitis

This inflammation of the iris, ciliary body, or choroid can be caused by a local infection or an immune response secondary to a systemic disorder (e.g., Crohn's disease), although the cause often is unclear. Patients with uveitis have eye pain, photophobia, and often, decreased vision. The pupil usually is constricted. Ciliary flush (injection of vessels around the corneal limbus) generally is present. Slit-lamp examination may show anterior chamber inflammation ("cells and flare"). These patients should be referred urgently to an ophthalmologist. Use of steroid eye drops should be in accordance with an ophthalmologist.

Vision Usually Normal

Conjunctivitis

Conjunctivitis often presents with ocular discharge and itching, without decrease in vision, and with conjunctival inflammation on examination. These patients can be treated with sulfacetamide or erythromycin topically (available as drops or ointments) for 7 days. Two notable exceptions to this are *herpetic conjunctivitis*, which also involves the cornea, with dendritic ulcers seen on fluorescein examination, and requires an immediate ophthalmologic consultation and admission; and *gonococcal conjunctivitis*, which usually produces profuse, purulent exudate and requires systemic treatment with penicillin along with topical antibiotics.

Corneal Abrasions and Foreign Bodies

These injuries can produce pain, itching, or a foreign-body sensation in the eye, without visual compromise. The patient may give a history of mild trauma to the eye. Be sure that there is no perforation of the globe. **PEARL: If the history includes the use of power tools or hitting metal with metal, obtain x-rays of the globe to exclude the presence of a metallic foreign body.**

PEARL: Irrigate all eyes with a sensation of a foreign body, even if you can't find one. Evert the eyelids because foreign bodies often get lodged underneath them. Fluorescein reveals the extent of the corneal lesion. In the past, these patients often had their eyes patched, but this probably is not necessary for either healing or comfort. Corneal abrasions resulting from contact lenses should not be patched. We usually give patients with corneal abrasions antibiotic ointment to apply four times a day to the eye, and we instruct them to return if they are not better within 24 hours. **PEARL: Avoid eye patching in patients with soft contact lenses.** All affected patients should receive tetanus prophylaxis as indicated (see Chapter 15). Table 8–1 summarizes the differential diagnosis of the red eye.

ACUTE VISUAL LOSS

PEARL: With severe acute visual loss, an afferent pupillary defect (APD) is usually present. When swinging a flashlight from one eye to the other, the pupil in the diseased eye di-

Table 8–1. DIFFERENTIAL DIAGNOSIS OF THE RED EYE

History and Clinical Findings	Conjunctivitis	Iritis	Acute Glaucoma	Corneal Infection (Bacterial Ulcer)	Corneal Ulcer
Incidence	Very common	Common	Common	Common	Common
Onset	Insidious	Insidious	Sudden	Slow	Sudden
Vision	Normal	Slightly blurred	Markedly blurred	Usually blurred	Blurred
Pain	None to moderate	Moderate	Severe	Moderate to severe	Severe
Photophobia	None to mild	Severe	Minimal	Variable	Moderate
Nausea and vomiting	None	None	Occasional	None	None
Discharge	Moderate to copious	None	None	Watery	Watery

Ciliary injection	Absent	Present, cir-cumcorneal	Present	Present	Present
Conjunctival injection	Severe, diffuse	Minimal	Minimal	Moderate	Mild
Cornea	Clear	Clear	Steamy	Hazy	Hazy
Stain with fluorescein	Absent	Absent	Absent	Present	Present
Hypopyon	Absent	Occasional	Absent	Occasional	Absent
Pupil size	Normal	Constricted	Midposition, fixed	Normal	Normal
Intraocular pressure	Normal	Normal	Elevated	Normal	Normal
Pupillary light response	Normal	Poor	None	Normal	Normal

lates when exposed to light due to a consensual response when the normal eye is no longer exposed to light. Acute binocular vision loss almost always indicates involvement of the CNS, specifically problems with the vertebrobasilar circulation. Therefore, in a patient presenting with sudden blindness, your workup should proceed as for a patient with a stroke or TIA (see Chapter 7). Note that some patients with migraine headaches can experience associated visual loss. Unless they give a history of temporary visual loss associated with their migraines, consider other diagnoses. Consider migraine to be a diagnosis of exclusion. In all patients with new binocular blindness, ophthalmologic consultation is mandatory. **PEARL: Acute visual loss is an emergency, and the affected patient should be seen by an ophthalmologist.**

Monocular visual loss can be due to either eye disorders or CNS problems. Patients with vision loss resulting from CNS causes can present with hemianopsia rather than monocular blindness. True monocular vision loss directs you to look for problems at the eye or optic nerve. The specific disorders you are likely to encounter are optic neuritis or neuropathy, retinal detachment, vitreous hemorrhage, and central retinal artery occlusion. In all of these cases, ophthalmologic consultation is mandatory. In some cases, emergency therapy is required.

Optic Nerve Disease

Most commonly called optic neuritis, optic nerve disease causes *visual loss and pain* behind the affected eye. About 30% of patients with optic neuritis develop multiple sclerosis (MS). It is now generally accepted that the standard of care for optic neuritis is admission for IV glucocorticoid therapy to reduce the patient's likelihood of developing MS.

Retinal Detachment

Retinal detachment can occur after trauma or in patients predisposed to retinal hemorrhage, such as diabetic patients or patients with coagulopathies. Monocular painless loss of vision is accompanied by a "shadow" or "curtain" sensation coming down over the affected eye. The detachment may not be visualized easily with the direct ophthalmoscope, so if you suspect this diagnosis, call the ophthalmologist. Therapy involves laser "tacking" of the retina.

Vitreous Hemorrhage

Vitreous hemorrhage is most commonly seen in diabetic patients and in patients with bleeding disorders. It involves bleeding into the vitreous chamber. You will most likely only see a red haze on funduscopy.

Giant Cell Arteritis

Also known as temporal arteritis, giant cell arteritis typically presents in patients older than 50 years. It is associated with headache, jaw claudication, visual loss, and a markedly elevated erythrocyte sedimentation rate (ESR). Polymyalgia rheumatica also may be present. A temporal artery may be tender. High-dose oral corticosteroids (e.g., prednisone, 60 mg per day) must be started to try to prevent visual loss in the other eye even before performing a definite temporal artery biopsy.

Central Retinal Artery Occlusion

Central retinal artery occlusion can be caused by cholesterol emboli, thrombotic embôli, or vasculitis. It is much more common in elderly patients, who have a much higher incidence of carotid atherosclerotic disease. The retina appears pale, with the macula looking like a cherry-red spot in the whitish-yellow background. You may see blood stains ("box-carring") or even the embolus itself. Begin treatment immediately; your goal is to lower the intraocular pressure to force the embolus more peripherally and perhaps, to preserve retinal tissue:

1. Give mannitol 1 g/kg IV and acetazolamide 500 mg IV to reduce production of aqueous humor.
2. Apply beta-blockers or pilocarpine eye drops.
3. "Ballot" the eye by applying intermittent pressure to the eyeball for 15 seconds out of every minute ("CPR of the eyeball").
4. Obtain an ophthalmologic consultation immediately to maximize the chances of vision salvage.

Central retinal *vein* occlusion occurs in the same age group as does central retinal artery occlusion and also causes monocular painless visual loss. Funduscopic examination reveals a blood-streaked retina. Even though no specific treatment exists, immediate consultation also is required.

OTHER EYE EMERGENCIES

Penetrating Eye Injuries

Although sometimes obvious, penetrating eye injuries may not always be apparent, especially when they involve the posterior part of the eye. A teardrop-shaped pupil suggests eye penetration with herniation of the iris through the wound. Visual acuity is often reduced, and the globe is soft. The eye should be protected with a rigid eye shield. The base of a plastic or styrofoam cup can be used to protect the eye from protrusion in the absence of a metal shield. The patient also should receive IV antibiotics (cefazolin 1 g and gentamicin 1.5 mg/kg) while waiting to see the ophthalmologist.

Chemical Burns of the Eyes

Chemical burns, especially alkali burns that cause liquefaction necrosis, can result in major tissue destruction. Immediate irrigation with 1 to 2 liters normal saline should be performed. Larger volumes of irrigant may be required to return the pH in the eye to normal. Irrigation can be facilitated by using a topical anesthetic to relieve the pain and any blepharospasm. It is helpful to check the pH of the eye 5 minutes after irrigation to ensure that a physiologic pH has been attained.

9
CHAPTER

ENT and Dental Emergencies

PREHOSPITAL CONSIDERATIONS

▶ Upper airway obstruction may be the most acute and most difficult medical emergency for EMS personnel.

▶ If the patient is choking but breathing, leave him or her alone to "cough it up." If his or her airway is obstructed, most people hold the hand across the front of the throat in the "universal choke" sign.

▶ Ask, "Can you speak?" If the patient is unable to answer, apply the Heimlich maneuver. If the patient falls unconscious, do abdominal thrusts.

▶ Always give 100% oxygen.

▶ For a patient with an acute nosebleed, pinch the nose together and hold for at least 15 minutes. Have the patient lean forward to prevent blood from dripping down the back of the throat.

▶ Never blindly stick anything in the patient's nose, ear, or throat to get out a foreign body; doing that usually pushes it in deeper.

DENTAL EMERGENCIES

Toothaches and mouth pain are very common complaints in the ED. Some institutions have a dentist on call;

most institutions do not. It falls upon the emergency medicine physician to deal with the acute problem. Start with the H&P. Most toothaches result from long-term neglect of dental caries. Therefore, when a patient comes to the ED, distinguish the conditions that need only analgesia from the more serious conditions. **PEARL: Not all toothaches are due to dental caries. Watch for the adult patient who complains of jaw pain radiating to the teeth and who may be having an acute myocardial infarction.**

Guidelines for the evaluation and treatment of a patient who appears to have a dental emergency include:

- Note whether the patient has a history of fever, facial swelling, pain to a specific tooth, or referred pain.
- Examine the mouth, lips, gums, and floor of the mouth. Tap on each tooth with a tongue blade to test sensitivity.
- Check for lesions, ulcers, blisters, vesicles, and any bleeding.
- Test for a possible salivary duct stone by milking the salivary glands.
- If there is any sign of an abscess, infection, pulpitis, gingivitis, or pericoronitis (infected impacted wisdom tooth), treat with appropriate analgesics and antibiotics.

Penicillin V (Penagen VK) and erythromycin cover most oral flora. Severe pain and a foul odor occurring several days after a tooth extraction may be the result of a dry socket. This is treated by irrigating the socket and applying iodoform gauze packing dampened by eugenol, followed by a dental referral.

Dental fractures with exposure of dentin (yellow appearing) should be covered with a calcium hydroxide–impregnated dressing and aluminum foil, with avoidance of exposure to extreme temperatures. If the tooth pulp is exposed (recognized by oozing of a drop of blood), immediate referral to a dentist or oral surgeon is preferred.

All avulsed teeth should be accounted for. **PEARL: Consider a chest x-ray to exclude aspiration when missing teeth cannot be accounted for.** Avulsed teeth may also become lodged in the soft tissues of the lips. Baby teeth should not be replaced, but avulsed permanent teeth should be replanted into the socket within the first 2 to 3 hours. This may require irrigation of the socket to remove any blood clots. Stabilization of the replanted tooth should be performed by a dentist as soon as possible.

EPIGLOTTITIS

As more and more children become appropriately immunized against *Haemophilus influenzae* (one of the most common infecting microbes), fewer cases of epiglottitis are being seen. In fact, the only cases of epiglottitis we have seen in the last 6 years have been in adults. Adults between 30 and 70 years old are most at risk. Epiglottitis may occur at any time in any season and is caused by a variety of microbes, burns, trauma, and other medical conditions. Besides *H. influenzae*, *Streptococcus pneumoniae* is a very common infecting microbe.

PEARL: Suspect acute epiglottitis in patients complaining of the worst sore throat of their life with few or no physical findings. Most often, there is no pharyngeal redness, and clinicians with less experience may believe that the patient is overreacting. Changes in the quality of the patient's voice are also common. For example, the patient may sound as if he or she is holding a "hot potato" in the throat and has severe pain with swallowing. These patients may have an immediate risk for airway obstruction.

There is controversy about the safety of direct visualization of the larynx in a patient with epiglottitis. If the patient is in respiratory distress or has signs and symptoms of imminent airway compromise, call for immediate ENT consultation and prepare for definitive airway management in the OR. If the patient presents with dysphagia and odynophagia, then careful direct fiberoptic laryngoscopy should be done to confirm the diagnosis. A lateral soft tissue x-ray of the neck may also be performed. The presence of a swollen epiglottis is suggested by a thumbprint-like appearance. Lack of a vallecular recess may also indicate epiglottitis (see Chapter 13). Once the diagnosis is made, be prepared to manage an acute airway obstruction. Despite this urgency, opinion is divided on whether to prophylactically intubate all patients with epiglottitis. **PEARL: Any patient having airway compromise should be intubated immediately.** Patients with minimal symptoms must be observed closely for signs of airway compromise. Death from epiglottitis is preventable with intubation.

UPPER AIRWAY OBSTRUCTION

The scariest situation that a patient experiences is the feeling of an impending airway obstruction. Airway management of these patients epitomizes the role of the emergency physician. Anticipation of a complete airway obstruction is necessary to avoid disaster. Most patients experience a gradual progression of airway obstruction, except in the settings of a foreign body or trauma.

Presentation

Patients with *complete upper airway obstruction* present with hoarseness, aphonia, tachypnea, tachycardia, severe agitation, stridor, and retraction of the supraclavicular and intercostal muscles, leading to cyanosis and loss of consciousness. This picture is very dramatic and may occur in a patient whom you are observing in the ED with a partial upper airway obstruction.

The presentation of a patient with a *partial upper airway obstruction* is less dramatic and is dominated by stridor and hoarseness with supraglottal obstruction, and wheezing and coughing with subglottal obstructions.

A short concise H&P may be all that time will allow for patients with an airway obstruction. They should be given 100% oxygen with continuous cardiac monitoring and pulse oximetry. X-rays should be done to rule out any foreign bodies.

Causes and Treatment

The most common cause of an upper airway obstruction is a *foreign body*, which, when lodged in the supraglottal space, will be amenable to the Heimlich maneuver. Small children can aspirate small objects that lodge in the subglottic space. This can be worsened by back blows or other similar maneuvers.

Other causes of upper airway obstruction are trauma, infections, hypersensitivity reactions, hemorrhage, and tumors. Most of these causes produce an insidious onset of airway compromise, which may need immediate attention in the ED.

Ludwig's angina, an infection and cellulitis of the floor of the mouth, can quickly obstruct the airway. This infection is usually associated with fever, pain on protrusion and elevation of the tongue, dysphagia, and trismus. The marked edema of the sublingual and submandibular spaces bulges the upper neck. Infection can spread to the mediastinum, causing a fatal mediastinitis. **PEARL: Patients with upper airway obstruction need immediate airway management, which may require tracheostomy, and high-dose penicillin, cephalosporin, or clindamycin therapy.** It is important to prepare for a difficult intubation along with cricothyroidotomy or tracheostomy or both. Immediate ENT consultation is usually necessary. It is uncommon for Ludwig's angina to have a drainable abscess; therefore, surgical incision and drainage are rarely indicated.

Patients who have *coagulation defects* or are on *warfarin* may have a similar presentation with hemorrhage into the floor of the mouth. Anaphylaxis may present as sudden onset of laryngeal edema and cause a sudden upper airway obstruction. These patients should be treated with subcutaneous epinephrine (1:1000) 0.01 mg/kg, diphenhydramine 50 mg IV, cimetidine 300 mg IV, and methylprednisolone 125 mg IV. Orotracheal intubation or cricothyrotomy may also be required.

Hereditary angioneurotic edema (angioedema) is an autosomal dominant condition that is manifested by sudden edema of the face, abdomen, and airway. This condition is most commonly characterized by a C1 esterase inhibitor deficiency. Affected patients should be treated similarly to those with allergic angioedema, as noted in the previous paragraph, with the addition of oral danazol 400 to 600 mg in two to three divided doses per day. Danazol increases the hepatic synthesis of C1 esterase inhibitor.

EPISTAXIS

Nosebleeds are a very common cause of emergency visits. They are classified as either anterior or posterior bleeds. Anterior bleeds are usually visible with a proper nasal examination. **PEARL: Prepare the nose with proper topical anesthesia and vasoconstriction, and thoroughly examine the nose for the site of a bleed.** It is often a visible anterior bleed. These nosebleeds may be very profuse because of their arterial origin, the Kiesselbach plexus. Therefore, patients may vomit blood when it drips down into the throat.

Most nosebleeds are the result of local trauma, such as self-exploration, cocaine, or upper respiratory infection, but they may be secondary to physical causes, such as coagulopathies, hepatic disease, or atherosclerosis. Posterior bleeds cannot be visualized and are more severe than anterior bleeds. **PEARL: If adequate tamponade of the anterior nose does not stop the bleeding, suspect a posterior source.**

Management

Most anterior nosebleeds can be controlled with proper preparation and equipment.

- Control the bleeding with external compression and soaked pledgets with equal parts of 4% viscous lidocaine and 1/4% to 1/2% phenylephrine (Neo-Synephrine) solution. If the bleeding source can be seen, apply a silver nitrate stick to cauterize the spot.
- The nose may be packed with 1 to 2 nasal tampons or, rarely, with a long strip of petroleum-impregnated gauze (Fig. 9–1).
- After the nose is packed, give prophylactic antibiotics or a first-generation cephalosporin (or augmentin) to reduce risk of staphylococcal toxic shock syndrome and acute sinusitis.
- The packing should remain for 3 to 5 days with the patient followed up by an ENT specialist. Premature removal of the nasal packing may result in recurrent bleeding.

If the bleeding continues or you cannot find the bleeder, the patient most likely has a posterior bleed. New combined anterior and posterior nasal devices that allow tamponade of both anterior and posterior portions of the nose are commercially available. **PEARL: Patients with posterior bleeds always require hospital admission and ENT consultation.** A posterior pack may be applied by using a Foley catheter or similar device into the nose, inflating the balloon and applying traction on the nasopharynx. This, combined with anterior packing, usually controls the bleeding.

Many patients experience an elevation in blood pressure during the course of treatment. Such patients may†be significantly hypovolemic (from bleeding), with resultant vasoconstriction, and should *not* be given a diuretic to lower their blood pressure. This results in worsening hypovolemia and may precipitate shock. Treatment with fluid hydration and control of the nasal bleeding is usually sufficient to treat the hypertension.

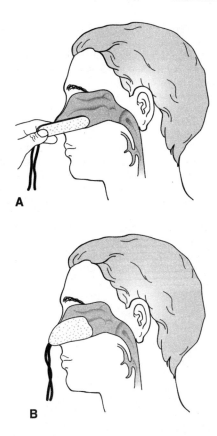

Figure 9–1. (*A*) After application of a topical anesthetic, the sponge packing should be lubricated with an antibiotic and gently inserted in the nasal cavity. (*B*) After the sponge is placed, it should be hydrated with normal saline, leading to its expansion.

NASAL FRACTURES

Nasal fractures should be suspected in any patient with facial trauma. A fracture is most likely due to a direct blow from an altercation, sports injury, or motor vehicle accident. Most patients have a tender ecchymotic area to the nose and, if soft tissue swelling is present, marked deformity. A simple, nondisplaced fracture of the nasal bone does not require any specific treatment other than analgesia. The patient should be referred to a plastic or ENT surgeon after the swelling has subsided, within 2 to 5 days. **PEARL: Nasal fractures usually don't require emergency treatment except when the patient has a septal hematoma or a cribiform plate fracture.**

- It is imperative to check the patient for *septal hematoma,* a rare complication caused by blood under the perichondrium of the nasal septum. If found, this hematoma should be gently incised with a #11 blade, drained, and packed to prevent the formation of an abscess or avascular necrosis of the septum (Fig. 9–2).

- Also look for signs of a CSF leak from a *fracture of the cribiform plate.* This is best done by means of metrizamide CT demonstrating extracranial CSF extravasation. **PEARL: CSF rhinorrhea cannot reliably be tested with filter paper and a ring test or a glucose test kit, but requires a head CT to rule out a cribiform plate fracture.** Such patients require immediate neurosurgical consultation.

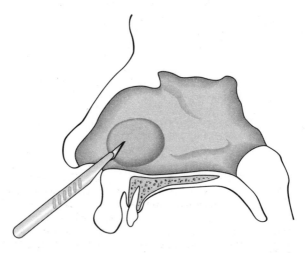

Figure 9–2. After applying a topical anesthetic supplemented with local infiltration, use a #11 surgical blade to make a small horizontal incision through the septal mucosa and perichondrium covering the hematoma.

FOREIGN BODIES

Most aural and nasal foreign bodies occur in children and vary in size and type. The most common foreign body in the ear is insects, especially roaches; in the nose, toys and plastic beads are most commonly found. It is always best to try to remove the foreign body with as minimal trauma as possible.

Ear

Patients with a foreign body in the ear may present with a painful draining ear, especially young children who may not verbalize the presence of a foreign body. Removal of the foreign body may be difficult because of poor patient cooperation. The examiner may have only one opportunity to use an instrument on the sensitive external canal. Where there is a partial blockage of the canal, irrigating with warm water behind the foreign body may successfully dislodge the object. Occasionally, an alligator forceps or a suction catheter may be used successfully. Placing Krazy Glue on the tip of a cotton swab (Q-Tip) to adhere to the foreign body has been used. With live insects in the ear, the external canal should be filled with 2% lidocaine or immersion oil, which causes the insect to "jump" out of the ear. **PEARL: Avoid irrigation in the presence of vegetative matter, since this may cause swelling of the foreign body.**

If your attempts to remove the foreign body fail, the patient should be taken to the OR to be properly sedated for foreign body removal with a binocular microscope. Repeated attempts in an uncooperative patient cause more harm than good.

Nose

Foreign bodies to the nose are almost exclusively seen in young children and institutionalized patients. These patients can present with a foul-smelling discharge, bleeding, or nasal obstruction. Manage by carefully preparing the nose, as described in treating epistaxis, with proper anesthesia and vasoconstriction. Before using any instruments, it may be worth attempting to have the parent of the child blow the foreign body out of the child's nose, especially with smooth objects that completely occlude the nasal passage. This is accomplished by having the parent put his or her mouth over the child's mouth and occluding the unblocked naris as in mouth-to-mouth respiration. The parent should blow against the child's closed glottis, forcing the foreign body out of the nose. An alligator forceps, a hook, or a Fogarty catheter may be used to remove a foreign body from the nose. **PEARL: After removing a foreign body, always look for more.** Often, a foreign body cannot be successfully removed in the ED and requires an ENT specialist to remove it in the OR.

OTALGIA

The most common cause of otalgia is an infection in the middle or external ear; however, other distant sources of earache can be remembered by the 5 Ts: throat, tonsils, temporomandibular joint, thyroid, and teeth. The pain from an ear infection may be severe enough to require narcotic analgesics.

Otitis Media

Otitis media is one of the most common diagnoses in the pediatric population. Tremendous controversy has arisen in the literature concerning the proper diagnosis and management of otitis media in children. The casual use of antibiotics in patients who "may have a red eardrum" is believed to be responsible for the increasing resistance of *S. pneumoniae* and other microbes to antibiotics. There is no gold standard for the diagnosis of otitis media; however, direct visualization of a reddened bulging tympanic membrane is the most commonly used criterion. Studies demonstrate that pneumatic testing for tympanic membrane mobility, either by hand or by electronic device, may enhance your sensitivity for the diagnosis. Tenderness over the mastoid process or anterior displacement of the ear suggests mastoiditis. This diagnosis should be confirmed with a head CT and requires urgent consultation with an ENT specialist.

Otitis Externa

Otitis externa is found in all age groups and is commonly associated with swimming—hence the term, "swimmer's ear." It can also be precipitated by sticking foreign objects into the ear, such as cotton-tip applicators and pencils. Here, the most common organism is *Pseudomonas*, which may be severe in elderly, immunocompromised, or diabetic patients who develop malignant otitis externa. Often, the ear canal is extremely swollen and narrowed, and it may be difficult to visualize the tympanic membrane. Pain on manipulation of the tragus and the auricle, however, clearly demonstrates the presence of otitis externa.

Treatment

Treatment of patients with otitis externa includes cleaning the ear canal and applying an ear wick so that topical analgesics and antibiotic solutions can penetrate into the ear canal. If there is any concern of a tympanic rupture due to the presence of discharge, use neomycin with corticosteroid suspension over solution. If you are unable to determine a concomitant otitis media, then oral antibiotics should be prescribed as well.

10
CHAPTER

Low Back Pain

Most people suffer from back pain sometime in their life, and it is considered one of the most common presentations in the ED. Although it has many causes, low back pain (LBP) usually is the result of benign conditions, and most patients respond to conservative treatment. **PEARL: Most patients with low back pain have a benign condition, but it is essential to diagnose the potentially serious condition, that is, spinal cord compression or AAA (abdominal aortic aneurysm).** In 1994, the Agency for Health Care Policy and Research (AHCPR) published guidelines regarding the assessment of adults 18 years of age and older with low back pain. The Internet address to obtain them is http://www.ahcpr.gov/. Once there, click on "Clinical Practice Guidelines" for a library of all of the guidelines issued to date.

Your job is to identify patients with serious, life-threatening, underlying diseases, such as vascular, abdominal, urinary, or pelvic conditions. Be especially diligent at the extremes of age. Children rarely complain of LBP, so assume it has a serious cause. Moreover, the elderly often have serious underlying conditions. **PEARL: Patients over 65 and children usually have organic disorders relating to their back pain.**

AHCPR GUIDELINES

- The initial assessment of patients with acute low back problems should focus on the detection of "red flags" (indicators of potentially serious spinal pathology or other nonspinal pathology).
- In the absence of red flags, imaging studies and further testing of patients are not usually helpful during the first 4 weeks of low back symptoms.
- Relief of discomfort can be accomplished most safely with nonprescription NSAID medications and/or spinal manipulation.
- Although some activity modification may be necessary during the acute phase, bed rest greater than 4 days is not helpful and may further debilitate the patient.
- Low-stress aerobic activities can be safely started in the first 2 weeks of symptoms to help avoid debilitation; exercises to condition trunk muscles are commonly delayed at least 2 weeks.
- Patients recovering from acute low back problems are encouraged to return to work or their normal activities as soon as possible.
- If low back symptoms persist, further evaluation may be indicated.
- Patients with sciatica may recover more slowly, but further evaluation can also be safely delayed.
- Within the first 3 months of low back symptoms, only patients with evidence of serious spinal pathology or severe debilitating symptoms of sciatica and with physiologic evidence of specific nerve root compromise corroborated on imaging studies can be expected to benefit from surgery.
- With or without surgery, 80% of patients with sciatica eventually recover.

HISTORY

The red flags outlined in the guidelines focus on the detection of traumatic or pathologic fractures, infections, or tumors of the spine. **PEARL: A complete history looking for indicators of serious pathology will help guide the seriousness of the condition.** The following suggest serious pathologic conditions:

1. Recent significant trauma.
2. Recent mild trauma in those over 50 years.
3. History of prolonged steroid use.
4. History of osteoporosis.
5. Patient age over 70 years.
6. History of cancer.
7. History of a recent infection.
8. Fever over 100° F.
9. IV drug use.
10. Low back pain worse at rest.
11. Unexplained weight loss.

The goal of the H&P is to classify the back pain into one of three categories:

- Potentially serious condition—tumor, infection, vascular pathology, fracture, or major neurologic compromise (e.g., cauda equina syndrome, AAA).
- Sciatica—symptoms suggesting nerve root compression.
- Nonspecific back symptoms—back pain without signs or symptoms suggesting sciatica or a potentially serious spinal condition.

Obtain the history with a series of open-ended questions such as "What are your symptoms?" Follow with more specific queries as to the presence of pain, numbness, weakness, stiffness, and so on. Urinary or bowel incontinence or retention should suggest spinal cord compression.

PHYSICAL EXAMINATION

Observe the patient before he or she realizes that you have begun your assessment. Often, the posture and facial expression change dramatically as soon as you enter the room. If possible, have the patient stand up; note how easy it is for him or her to get up. Look at the patient's back. Are there any obvious deformities (scoliosis or kyphosis)? Is there evidence of trauma? Palpate the length of the spinal column, paravertebral musculature, buttocks, and flanks for areas of tenderness. Have the patient point to the area of maximal discomfort. Have the patient stand and test to see how far forward he or she can bend at the waist. An increase in pain with flexion may suggest a disk problem. Assessing range of motion is, however, very subjective and may not always be helpful (although severe guarding of lumbar motion in all planes is more likely to support a diagnosis of an infection, tumor, or fracture).

Ask the patient to walk on the heels (this tests foot dorsiflexion) and on the toes (this tests foot plantar flexion). Next, have the patient sit on the edge of the examining table to assess for deep tendon reflexes (if you don't have a reflex hammer, you can use the head of your stethoscope). Test the ankle (S_1) and knee (L_3, L_4) reflexes in both legs. Many patients do not have good reflexes. Distracting the patient can help elicit deep tendon reflexes. While the patient is still sitting, listen for breath sounds and auscultate the heart. (In rare cases, a pneumothorax may present as sudden onset of sharp pleuritic back pain.)

Have the patient lie supine and examine the abdomen for a pulsating mass (aortic aneurysm), hepatomegaly, or discrete masses (may suggest malignancy). Listen for abdominal or flank bruits. Check for femoral and pedal pulses. Women require a full pelvic examination unless the cause of their back pain is readily apparent. Pay particular attention to the presence of fever, lymphadenopathy, or any needle "track marks."

Straight leg raising (SLR) tests for true sciatica, indicating a radicular origin of the pain. Passively flex the outstretched legs at the hip and see if, and at what level (expressed as degrees), pain shoots down the leg (Fig. 10–1). Back pain is not considered a positive finding. Helpful hints: Dorsiflexion of the foot increases true sciatica, whereas flexion at the knee decreases the pain elicited during SLR. Increased pain on raising the contralateral leg (crossed SLR) is even more specific for a radicular origin of the pain.

It may be difficult to determine whether there is a functional, nonorganic component of the patient's LBP. (Be aware, also, that most *chronic* LBP has a psychological component.) Helpful hints that suggest a functional disorder include the following:

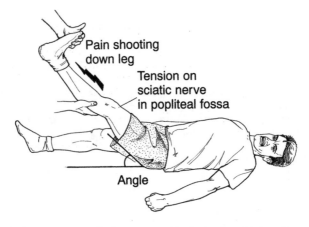

Figure 10–1. Straight leg raising eliciting pain, which radiates down the leg. The pain is exacerbated by dorsiflexing the foot and putting tension on the sciatic nerve in the popliteal fossa.

- Application of pressure to the top of the head is reported by the patient to increase LBP (with organic pathology, it should not).
- Hip or shoulder rotation is reported to increase LBP (it should not).
- Inconsistent findings in SLR when lying and sitting.
- Patient appears to be overreacting.

Spinal Cord Syndromes

Disease processes involving the spinal cord and its elements usually present as one of two symptom complexes:

1. **Radiculopathy** is due to pressure on spinal roots. Most often, only one or a few segmental levels are involved, and the patient presents with sharp segmental pain and loss of sensation and motor weakness at the corresponding level. If the muscle is involved in a deep tendon reflex arc, the reflex will be weak or absent.
2. **Myelopathy** is secondary to pressure on the spinal cord itself. The patient presents with partial or total loss of sensory and motor function below the level of the lesion.

THE NEUROLOGIC EXAMINATION

It is helpful to assess each of the three spinal cord sections separately:

1. The **anterior cord** is assessed by testing the gross motor function of various muscle groups and cord levels.
2. The **lateral cord** is assessed by testing for pinprick sensation or two-point discrimination.
3. The **posterior cord** is assessed by testing proprioception (sense of positioning), vibration sensation, or both. Have patients close their eyes and indicate whether you are pointing their big toe downward or upward.

Table 10–1 will help you to determine the level of the spinal lesion based on clinical findings.

Because most neurologic deficits result from disk herniation, and most herniations are at the level of L4–5 or L5–S1, particular emphasis should be placed on testing toe dorsiflexion and plantar flexion, sensation between the first and second toes and on the undersurface of the foot, and the presence or absence of an ankle jerk.

A rectal (perineal) examination and assessment for saddle anesthesia are always good ideas, but especially in the presence of the following:

- Any neurologic deficit.
- Symptoms of bowel or bladder dysfunction.
- A recent change in bowel habits or rectal bleeding.
- An elderly man in whom prostatic cancer is likely.

Table 10–1. DETERMINING THE LEVEL OF SPINAL INVOLVEMENT

Level of Lesion	Level of Sensory Loss	Motor Deficit	Lost Reflex
L1	Groin crease	Hip flexion	—
L2, L3	Medial thigh	Hip adduction	—
L4	Knee	Hip abduction	Patellar
L5	Lateral calf, first toe webspace	Foot and big toe dorsiflexion	—
S1	Lateral foot	Foot and big toe plantar flexion	Achilles
S2–S4	Perianal region	Rectal sphincter tone	—

ANCILLARY TESTS

In most patients, a detailed H&P is enough to rule out serious pathologic conditions, and no further tests are necessary except in the presence of red flags.

X-rays of the lumbosacral spine may be indicated in the following circumstances:

- Recent significant trauma.
- Evidence of malignant disease anywhere in the body.
- Age extremes (<18 years and >50 years).
- Unresolved back pain >30 days.
- Fever, weight loss, adenopathy, or signs of systemic illness.
- History of IV drug abuse or alcohol abuse.
- History of tuberculosis (Pott's disease).
- Neurologic deficits.

Significantly elevated *erythrocyte sedimentation* rate (ESR) or *WBCs* suggests metastatic disease, infectious disease, or inflammatory disease.

If you suspect renal calculi or infection, perform a dipstick or full *urinalysis*. **PEARL: Remember that a normal urinalysis result does not exclude nephrolithiasis.**

In patients older than 50 years with lower flank or back pain, especially if they are hypotensive, consider performing an immediate bedside *ultrasound* to exclude an abdominal aortic aneurysm.

ACUTE SPINAL CORD COMPRESSION

Spinal cord compression is a medical emergency requiring urgent surgical decompression or radiation therapy.

Patients with spinal cord compression can present with loss of sensation and motor function below the level of compression and with some degree of bowel and/or bladder dysfunction. The causes of acute cord compression include:

- **Tumors:** primary or secondary (e.g., lung, breast, prostate, lymphoma, multiple myeloma).
- **Infections:** epidural abscess.
- **Trauma:** dislocation of the vertebra or vertebral body collapse.
- **Disk injury:** ruptured intervertebral disk or severe central herniation or compression.
- **Spinal cord hematoma:** spontaneous or traumatic.

Often, there is segmental involvement of spinal roots at the level of the lesion, and the patient presents with unilateral or bilateral pain radiating in a dermatomal pattern or with radicular parasthesias. All patients with acute spinal cord compression need immediate admission and a workup that includes plain films of the spine (look for vertebral body collapse, bony erosions, or paraspinal soft tissue masses) and MRI (or CT scanning with metrizamide myelography).

All patients should be immobilized adequately before you proceed with any diagnostic or therapeutic measures. For patients with traumatic spinal cord injuries, give an IV bolus of methylprednisolone 30 mg/kg within 8 hours of injury, followed by 5.4 mg/kg per hour over the next 23 hours.

DISPOSITION

Most patients with LBP, even in the presence of stable isolated neurologic deficits, can be sent home safely. Indications for hospital admission include:
- Acute spinal cord compression
- Serious underlying diseases (e.g., abdominal or thoracic aneurysm)
- Spinal cord infections
- Intractable pain (rarely the sole indication)
- Multiple nerve root involvement
- Progressive or severe neurologic impairment
- Unstable fractures, traumatic dislocations, or subluxation
- Acute spinal trauma and neurologic deficits

MANAGEMENT

Initial care of the patient with nonspecific back pain consists of assurance and education, measures to provide patient comfort, and advice regarding alteration of activities. If the initial assessment detects no serious condition, assure the patient that "there is no hint of a dangerous problem" and that "a rapid recovery can be expected." Patients with sciatica may have a longer expected recovery period than those with nonspecific back pain and thus, may need more assurance and education.

NSAIDs or *acetaminophen* provide sufficient pain relief for most patients with acute low back pain, with acetaminophen being considered the safest of these. Although NSAIDs can be effective, potential risks include gastrointestinal, renal, and allergic manifestations. Acetaminophen may be used safely in combination with NSAIDs, especially in otherwise well patients, according to the panel's assessment. The new COX-2 inhibitors (e.g., Vioxx 12.5 to 50 mg once daily) may also be considered, especially in patients at risk for gastrointestinal bleeding (e.g., the elderly). Muscle relaxants are felt to be no more effective than NSAIDs for treating low back symptoms, and using them in conjunction with NSAIDs has no demonstrated benefit.

Opioids appear to be no more effective than safer analgesics in patients with LBP, and it is felt that they generally should be avoided in the treatment of back pain. When necessary, they should be used for a short time only. Your least concern should be an addictive effect.

Physical modalities such as massage, diathermy, ultrasound, cutaneous laser treatment, biofeedback, and transcutaneous electrical nerve stimulation have no proven efficacy in the treatment of acute low back pain. Self-application of heat or cold may provide some temporary symptomatic relief. *Invasive techniques* such as needle acupuncture and injection procedures (trigger points or facets with steroids and/or lidocaine) have no proven benefit in the treatment of acute low back pain. In addition, corsets and back belts do not appear to be beneficial.

Most patients do not require bedrest, and prolonged rest (more than 4 days) can have debilitating effects and its efficacy is unproven. To avoid debilitation, patients should perform aerobic activities such as walking, use of a stationary bicycle, swimming, and even light jogging. There is no evidence that back-specific exercise machines are effective for treating low back problems or evidence that stretching the back alleviates symptoms. Acute limitations of work duties may be appropriate. Make it clear to both patients and their employers that even moderately heavy unassisted lifting may aggravate back symptoms and restrictions are intended to allow spontaneous recovery or time to build activity tolerance through exercise.

PROGNOSIS

Within 6 weeks, 90% of episodes of acute LBP respond to treatment or resolve spontaneously. Although approximately 5% of patients will require admission, only 1% require surgery. Patients should be instructed to return to the ED if they develop any bladder or bowel dysfunction or progressive muscle weakness in the legs.

PEARL: Never assume malingering or that nothing is wrong. The patient's pain is always real to the patient.

11
CHAPTER

Poisonings and Principles of Toxicology

PREHOSPITAL CONSIDERATIONS

▸ Before leaving the scene, prehospital personnel should search the patient's belongings and surroundings for evidence of toxic agents.
▸ Vital functions should be supported by addressing the ABCs.
▸ Make sure that the patient has an established IV and is attached to a cardiac monitor and continuous oxygen supply.
▸ In patients with a depressed CNS, glucose, thiamine, and naloxone should be administered. Glucose may be withheld if a rapid glucose test is above 80 mg/dL.
▸ Rapid transport to the nearest medical facility is appropriate.

RECOGNIZING POISONINGS

The most important factor in determining the outcome in acute poisonings is early recognition that one is dealing with a toxicologic problem. Generally, it is wise to consider a poisoning in all patients presenting to the ED. In the following situations particularly, ask yourself whether the patient's condition is secondary to an acute or chronic poisoning:

- Altered mental status
- Abnormal vital signs not readily explained by other underlying pathology
- Anion gap metabolic acidosis
- Significant osmolar gap
- Depressed or suicidal patient
- Known history of overdose
- Children between the ages 1 and 5 years and 11 and 18 years
- Patient or family stating that the patient swallowed pills
- EMS personnel finding empty pill containers at the scene of injury
- Classic signs and symptoms of a toxidrome
- Psychiatric patients on medications
- Elderly patients on cardiac medications
- Unexplained illness after ingesting food, drink, or medication
- Many individuals with illnesses all beginning at the same time

Remember that in cases of poisoning the historic information obtained from bystanders may be inaccurate or even misleading. Always maintain a high index of suspicion.

Patients with poisonings can present with no symptoms at all. When toxicity is delayed, focus on preventing drug absorption and monitoring for evidence of toxicity. IV access, continuous cardiac monitoring, and frequent reevaluations are necessary in all patients with a potential poisoning.

In many situations, laboratory confirmation of a specific poison is not available in the ED. Initiation of both nonspecific and specific therapy must be based on your clinical judgment, with the degree of urgency dictated by the gravity of the patient's condition. Regional poison control centers can be invaluable sources of information.

INITIAL ASSESSMENT

All poisoning patients require a rapid assessment of their ABCs. **PEARL: Stabilize ABCs in all patients first.** Resuscitation and stabilization often are begun before any information is available. Don't let EMS personnel leave before you obtain as much information as possible concerning a potential overdose. If the EMS personnel are unsure, send them or the police back to the scene, if possible, to collect any evidence. **PEARL: Get history from other sources such as family, primary care physician, pharmacist, or the patient's physician.** The following are important questions to ask.

- What were the patient's vital signs and initial mental status at the scene?
- What therapy was given en route to the hospital?
- Was there any evidence of intoxication?
- Were any pill containers found?
- What medications were found? (Find out the names, strengths, and original and present number of pills.)
- Was there any possibility of exposure to environmental toxins? **PEARL: Have patients' belongings and dwelling searched for evidence of poisons and medications.**
- What is the patient's occupation?
- Where does the patient work?
- When did the overdose occur?
- Was ingestion intentional or accidental?
- When was the patient last seen?

Physical Examination

The physical examination assumes the utmost importance because it often elicits vital clues to the nature of the poisoning. Perform a detailed physical examination with particular emphasis on vital signs, neurologic examination, pupil response, skin, and diagnostic odors. A detailed list of effects of specific toxins on the various organ systems is presented in Appendix B. These exhaustive lists may be helpful, but a combination of signs and symptoms produced by a toxin or a category of toxins may be useful.

TOXIDROMES

PEARL: Look for toxidromes. Once you suspect a poisoning, try to determine whether the pattern of signs and symptoms fits into any particular toxidrome (toxic syndrome). The more common toxidromes are presented in Table 11–1. **PEARL: Remember that your local poison control center can be very helpful in the diagnosis and management of poisonings.** Many regions provide telephone assistance: 1-800-POISONS.

Table 11-1. COMMON TOXIDROMES

Toxidrome/Drug	Clinical Manifestations	Treatment
Anticholinergics Antihistamines, antispasmodics, atropine, benztropine, antiparkinsonian drugs, antipsychotics, antidepressants, cyclic antidepressants, phenothiazines, mydriatic agents, sleep medications, jimson weed	Tachycardia, tachypnea, hypertension, hyperthermia, seizures, hallucinations, delirium, mydriasis, flushed skin, decreased bowel sounds, thirst, urinary retention	Intravenous (IV) fluids, benzodiazepines (lorazepam 1–2 mg IV or IM q 10 min), antipyretics, physostigmine 1–2 mg IV (0.5 mg in children) for seizures or resistant dysrhythmias
Sympathomimetics Cocaine, amphetamine, PCP, LSD, phenylpropanolamine	CNS excitation, seizures, hypertension, tachycardia, mydriasis, tremors, diaphoresis, normal bowel sounds	IV fluids, benzodiazepines (lorazepam 1–2 mg IV or IM) q 10 min
Cholinergics Organophosphates, carbamates, edrophonium, mushrooms, pilocarpine, betel nut	**DUMBBELSS** or **SLUDGE:** defecation, urination, miosis, bradycardia, bronchospasm, emesis, lacrimation, secretions, seizures	Atropine 2 mg IV (0.05 mg/kg in children) q 10 min until no respiratory secretions; pralidoxime 1 g IV for organophosphates
Sedatives/hypnotics Heroin, morphine, codeine, propoxyphene, pentazocine, diphenoxylate, meperidine,	Hypoventilation, CNS depression, miosis (for most opioids except meperidine and diphenoxylate), hypotension	Oxygenation and ventilation, intravenous fluids, naloxone 0.4–2 mg IV, SC, IM, IT for

benzodiazepines, barbiturates, alcohols, chloral hydrate		opioid overdose, give lower doses and restrain in chronic abusers; flumazenil 1–3 mg IV (20–30 mg/kg/dose in children) for life threatening effects of isolated benzo-diazepine overdose
Withdrawal of substances of abuse Alcohol, opioids, barbiturates, chloryl hydrate	Tachycardia, diarrhea, vomiting, mydriasis, piloerection, lacrimation, yawning, agitation, seizures	Benzodiazepines (lorazepam 1–2 mg IV or IM q 10 min), neuroleptics (droperidol 2.5–5.0 mg IV or IM q 5–10 min)
Serotonin syndrome Fluoxetine, paroxetine, sertraline, fluvoxamine	Neurobehavioral manifestations (agitation, confusion, seizures), autonomic manifestations (hyperthermia, diaphoresis, diarrhea, tachycardia, hypertension, salivation), neuromuscular manifestations (rigidity, ataxia, tremor, hyperreflexia, ataxia, myoclonus)	Benzodiazepines (lorazepam 1–2 mg IV or IM q 10 min), IV fluids, ventilation, muscle relaxants, antipyretics, antidysrhythmic agents

CNS = central nervous system; **DUMBBELSS: D** = defecation, **U** = urination, **M** = miosis, **B** = bradycardia, **B** = bronchospasm, **E** = emesis, **L** = lacrimation, **S** = secretions, **S** = seizures; IM = intramuscularly; IT = intrathecally; LSD = lysergic acid; PCP = phencyclidine; SC = subcutaneously; **SLUDGE: S** = salivation; **L** = lacrimation; **U** = urination; **D** = defecation; **G** = gastrointestinal irritation; **E** = emesis.

INITIAL MANAGEMENT

Always start by assessing the patient's ABCs. Patients who are lethargic or unresponsive often need to be intubated to protect their airway. **PEARL: All patients with an altered mental status should receive the following treatment.**

1. **100% O$_2$** via a nonrebreather mask.
2. **Thiamine** 100 mg IV (should be given before glucose).
3. **Glucose** should be checked with a glucose oxidase indicator strip (Dextrostix, Ames Co., Elkhart, IN). If a glucose level is not immediately available or if it is < 60 to 80 mg/dL, give 50 mL D$_{50}$W IV push (2 to 4 mL D$_{25}$W/kg in children).
4. **Naloxone** 2 mg IV (0.1 mg/kg up to 2 mg in children). You may consider giving up to 20 mg IV, especially in the setting of propoxyphene, meperidine, or oxycodone overdose. Give less if there is the possibility of an acute withdrawal reaction. **PEARL: Patients with suspected opioid overdose or dependency should be physically restrained prior to administration of naloxone, since violent responses may occur.** Unresponsive patients with lateralizing signs should have an urgent head CT scan.

NONSPECIFIC THERAPY

The following treatment guidelines are aimed at decreasing the absorption and enhancing the elimination of potential toxins.

Gastric Decontamination

The role of gastric decontamination is still evolving. Both gastric lavage and activated charcoal are most effective when given within the first hour after ingestion of a toxin. The role of ipecac is even less clear and may be indicated only for toxic plant ingestion.

Activated Charcoal

Activated charcoal is probably the most effective decontaminant. It acts by adsorbing toxin present in the gastrointestinal tract. Even when gastric lavage is indicated, activated charcoal should be administered via the orotracheal tube before lavage. Adults should receive 50 to 100 g

PO (children 1 to 2 g/kg). Use the mnemonic CHARCOAL to remember substances that are *not* adsorbed by activated charcoal:

C caustics and corrosives
H heavy metals
A alcohols and glycols
R rapidly absorbed substances
C cyanide, chlorine
O other insoluble drugs
A aliphatic hydrocarbons
L laxatives

Other contraindications for the use of activated charcoal are absent bowel sounds or other signs of intestinal obstruction or perforation. Repeated doses of activated charcoal are indicated for the following poisonings: aspirin, carbamazepine, theophylline, phenobarbital, dapsone, and quinidine.

Gastric Lavage

Gastric lavage usually is effective only if performed within 30 to 60 minutes of toxic ingestion (it may still be effective if given later in intoxications with substances that slow down gastrointestinal motility, such as anticholinergic agents). Gastric lavage is probably even less effective than activated charcoal. It is indicated in patients with ingestion of toxic substances not adsorbed by activated charcoal, in patients with massive lethal doses of pills (especially if they can form concretions in the intestines), and in unstable patients in whom intubation is indicated. The patient should be placed in the left lateral position with the head lower than the hips. Use a large orogastric tube (36F to 40F in adults and 16F to 28F in children). Lavage should never be performed in patients with actual or potential mental obtundation or seizures without prior protection of the airway with a cuffed endotracheal tube. (Cuffed tubes are not appropriate in children younger than 6 years.) Lavage with aliquots of 250 mL NS (50 to 100 mL in children) until gastrointestinal contents are clear. Attach a 60-mL syringe (whose plunger has been removed) to the tube, and pour NS directly into the syringe; then drain, using gravity or low suction (Fig. 11–1). An oral airway may be placed between the teeth to prevent the patient

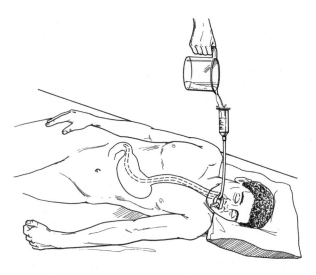

Figure 11–1. Gastric lavage. The patient is placed in the left lateral position with the head down.

from biting down on the tube when awakening or having a seizure. Before removal, pinch off the tube to avoid dripping fluid down into the airway. *Absolute contraindications to gastric lavage include:*

- Caustic ingestions
- Intestinal obstruction
- Intestinal perforation
- Age < 9 months

Ipecac

Although possibly useful in the home setting, ipecac is rarely indicated in the ED. Ipecac may be given to patients with recent (within 30 minutes) mushroom or unknown plant ingestions in which gastric lavage would be ineffective. Adults should receive 30 to 60 mL PO; children > 15 months, 15 mL PO; and children < 15 months, 10 mL PO. Avoid giving ipecac to any patient with the potential for rapid deterioration of mental status (e.g., those who have ingested cyclic antidepressants) or development of seizures. Other contraindications include ingestion of corrosives, caustics, petroleum distillates, or foreign bodies; loss of the gag reflex; hemodynamic unstability; age less than 6 months; and vomiting since ingestion of substance.

Cathartics

Many cathartics are available, but magnesium citrate is the most useful because of its palatability. (Avoid it if the patient is in renal failure because of the risk of hypermagnesemia.) Adults should receive 30 g PO (300 mL of 10% solution). Sorbitol is an alternate cathartic (give adults 40 mL of 70%). In acetaminophen poisoning, saline sulfate (15 to 30 g PO) is preferred because it can enhance the sulfate metabolic pathway and provide hepatic protection. Cathartics are contraindicated in gastrointestinal bleeding or ileus and should not be given to children younger than 2 years old.

Enhanced Elimination

Alkalinization of the urine is useful in eliminating weak acids such as salicylates and barbiturates. This is achieved with IV boluses of sodium bicarbonate 8.5% to maintain a urinary pH of 7.5 to 8.0.

Early dialysis may be required in the following poisonings: methyl alcohol, ethylene glycol, *Amanita phalloides* (a poisonous mushroom), aspirin, and lithium. Note that dialysis is most effective with water-soluble agents that have a low volume of distribution (< 1 L/kg), poor protein binding ($< 50\%$), and low molecular weights (usually < 600 d). Charcoal hemoperfusion can be indicated in theophylline overdose. Whole bowel irrigation has been shown to be useful in severe iron overdoses.

ANCILLARY TESTS IN ACUTE POISONINGS

Once you suspect an intoxication, the following lab tests should be ordered.

1. **Chem 7** (electrolytes, bicarbonate, glucose, BUN, and creatinine): This allows you to calculate the anion gap $[Na - (HCO_3 + Cl)]$, which helps sort out the various causes of metabolic acidosis (normally 10 ± 2). The following is a list of common causes of an anion gap metabolic acidosis (use the mnemonic **MUDPILES**):

M　methanol
U　uremia
D　diabetic ketoacidosis
P　propylene glycol, paraldehyde, phenformin
I　iron, isoniazide, inhalants (CO, CN, H_2S)
L　lactic acidosis (seizure, shock, hypoxia)
E　ethylene glycol, ethanol
S　salicylates, solvents (toluene)

A low anion gap suggests the presence of bromides, lithium, or abnormal cationic proteins.

2. **Analysis of ABGs** allows rapid assessment of the oxygenation status and the acid-base balance. Respiratory alkalosis can be an early manifestation of salicylate overdose. The differential diagnosis of acid-base abnormalities is presented in Chapter 2. Carboxyhemoglobin levels should be assessed rapidly if CO poisoning is suspected.

3. **Serum osmolarity:** Calculate the osmolar gap by subtracting the calculated osmolarity from the measured osmolarity. The calculated osmolarity should equal:

$$2\,Na + \frac{Glucose}{18} + \frac{BUN}{2.8} + \frac{Alcohol}{MW \div 10}$$

where MW = molecular weight of the alcohol.

Alcohols are the most common cause of an increased osmolar gap. Blood levels of the various alcohols can be estimated from the osmolar gap if their molecular weights are known (ethanol = 46; methanol = 32; ethylene glycol = 62; isopropanol = 60). Other causes of an osmolar gap include isoniazide, mannitol, and trichloroethane. Note, however, that measurements of osmolarity are not always accurate or helpful because of frequent laboratory error.

4. **Acetaminophen level:** Acetaminophen is the most commonly ingested toxin and frequently is a component of a combined overdose. Because there is a known antidote, it is cost-effective to include an acetaminophen level in the "tox labs." Acetaminophen levels should be obtained 4 hours after the ingestion. If the time of ingestion is unknown, it is useful to draw two blood levels at least 1 hour apart and to look for a trend in the levels. Repeating acetaminophen levels may also be helpful in cases of ingestion of long-acting preparations. The Rumack-Matthew nomogram, illustrated in Figure 11–2, is useful in predicting the probability of hepatic injury based on acetaminophen levels.

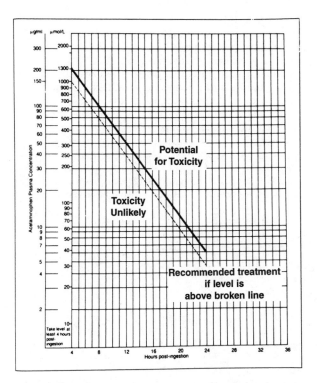

Figure 11–2. The Rumack-Matthew nomogram for acute single ingestion of acetaminophen. (Reproduced by permission of *Pediatrics*, vol. 55, p. 873, copyright 1975.)

5. **Salicylate level:** This, too, is a common primary or co-ingestant. Levels should be determined 6 hours after ingestion. A level over 30 mg/dL is considered toxic. Treatment never should be delayed if the patient is already symptomatic. The Done nomogram, although widely cited, is not always reliable.

6. **Plain abdominal films** can be helpful if you suspect the ingestion of a radiopaque material (use the mnemonic **CHIPES**):

   C chloral hydrate, cocaine condoms, calcium, chlorinated hydrocarbons

   H heavy metals (e.g., arsenic, lead)

    I   iron, iodides
    P phenothiazines, potassium, Pepto-Bismol, Play-Doh
    E enteric coated tablets
    S slow-release capsules, solvents

7. **Specific quantitative laboratory analysis** on an emergency basis should be obtained for the following agents: methanol, ethylene glycol, isopropyl alcohol, iron, theophylline, lithium, monoxide, digoxin, phenytoin, phenobarbital, and carbamazepine.

8. **Urinalysis:** Microscopic observation of rhomboid or needle-shaped calcium oxalate stones suggests ethylene glycol poisoning (Fig. 11–3). Observe the urine under a Wood's lamp. Fluorescence suggests the presence of antifreeze, a common source of ethylene glycol (also look

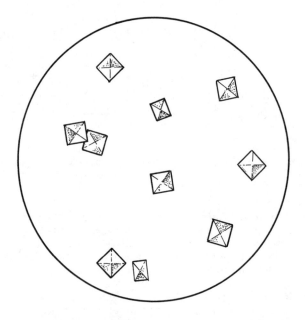

Figure 11–3. Calcium oxalate stones in the urine of a patient with ethylene glycol poisoning.

for fluorescence around the patient's mouth). If on adding several drops of 10% $FeCl_2$ the urine turns purple, suspect salicylate or phenothiazine poisoning. If the color blanches on adding 20% sulfuric acid, phenothiazines are more likely.

SPECIFIC POISONINGS

Although a detailed review of the clinical manifestations of all toxic substances is not possible here, highlights of a few of the more common or more lethal substances not already mentioned in the toxidromes section, as well as their specific treatment, are presented in Table 11–2.

DISPOSITION

Factors that will affect your decision regarding disposition include:

- Clinical manifestations: Symptomatic patients should be admitted for observation. Unstable patients should be admitted to a monitored unit.
- Pharmacokinetics of the specific toxin: The onset, peak action, and duration of the agent all must be taken into account. Obviously, if the time elapsed since the ingestion is greater than the duration of the ingested toxin, it is safe to discharge the asymptomatic patient.
- Suicidal or homicidal ideation: Any patient who continues to be a threat to him- or herself or others should be evaluated by a psychiatrist or admitted with constant observation.

All patients with a potentially serious overdose should be observed for at least 2 to 6 hours before discharge or transfer to a nonmedical unit.

Some of the delayed-reacting substances that require more than 6 hours of observation can be remembered by the mnemonic **WAIT**:

W warfarin
A acetonitrile
I industrial paint stripper (methylene chloride)
T toxic cyanogenic plants and serious mushroom poisonings

Table 11-2. COMMON INGESTIONS

Drug/Toxic Dose or Level	Clinical Manifestations	Treatment
Acetaminophen >7.5 g in adults (may be lower in alcoholics and starvation) >140 mg/kg in children See Figure 11–2 for toxic levels	May be asymptomatic despite serious ingestion; nausea, vomiting, abdominal pain, jaundice, confusion	*N*-acetylcysteine 140 mg/kg PO followed by 17 doses of 70 mg/kg PO q 4 h; repeat dose if vomited within 1 h; dilution in chilled fruit juice or addition of an antiemetic (metoclopramide 10 mg IV) may improve compliance
Salicylates 150–300 mg/kg: mild to moderate toxicity 300–500 mg/kg: severe toxicity >500 mg/kg: potentially lethal	Nausea, vomiting, hyperpnea, tinnitus, fever, disorientation, lethargy, coma, seizures, diaphoresis, abdominal pain, gastrointestinal (GI) bleeding, noncardiogenic pulmonary edema	IV fluids and frequent boluses of sodium bicarbonate 1 mEq/kg IV to maintain a urine output of 2–3 mL/kg/h and urine pH of 7.5–8.0; hemodialysis for severe cases and level >100 mg/dL
Cyclic antidepressants	CNS excitation, confusion, blurred vision, dry mouth fever, mydriasis, dysrhythmias, ECG QRS interval > 100 ms, ECG rightward axis terminal of 40 msec, hypotension, tachycardia, respiratory depression	IV fluids, frequent boluses of sodium bicarbonate 1–2 mEq/kg for QRS >100 ms, life-threatening dysrhythmias, or persistent hypotension
Theophylline >25–30 µg/mL	GI irritation, agitation, disorientation, seizures, dysrhythmias, hypokalemia,	Repeated dose of activated charcoal 0.5 g/kg q 2–4 h;

	hyperglycemia	standard treatment of seizures and dysrhythmias, hemodialysis or charcoal hemoperfusion for levels > 100 µg/mL (acute) or > 40 µg/mL (chronic)
Digoxin >2.5 ng/mL	GI irritation, delirium, visual disturbances, conduction blocks, dysrhythmias, hyperkalemia with normal renal function in acute toxicity	Atropine or pacemaker for bradydysrhythmias, phenytoin or lidocaine for tachydysrhythmias; digoxin-specific Fab fragments 10 ampules IV for potassium >5.5, resistant life-threatening dysrhythmias, and a digoxin level >10 ng/mL 6 h postingestion
Iron >20 mg/kg elemental iron >300–500 µg/dL: moderate toxicity >500 µg/dL: severe toxicity	GI bleeding, leukocytosis, hyperglycemia, metabolic acidosis, hepatic failure, shock, coma, late GI obstruction	Deferoxamine 15 mg/kg/h IV for symptomatic patients, ingestions >30 mg/kg, iron level >500 µg/dL, vin rose urine after deferoxamine challenge (50 mg/kg IM)
Carbon monoxide >10%	Simultaneous symptoms in household members, dyspnea, headache, confusion, tachycardia, tachypnea, coma, seizures,	100% O_2 via mask; hyperbaric O_2 for COHb >25% (COHb >15% in children, pregnant women,

Table continued on following page

Table 11-2. COMMON INGESTIONS *(Continued)*

Drug/Toxic Dose or Level	Clinical Manifestations	Treatment
	cherry red skin, retinal hemorrhages, metabolic acidosis	or patients with IHD), ECG changes, CNS symptoms, metabolic acidosis, combined COHb and cyanide overdose
Calcium channel blockers	Confusion, hypotension, bradycardia, atrioventricular blocks, seizures, respiratory depression, coma, cyanosis, hyperglycemia	IV fluids, atropine 0.5–1 mg IV q 5 min up to 3 mg, calcium chloride 1 g IV (20–30 mg/kg in children), catecholamine pressors, glucagon, pacing
Beta-blockers	Confusion, bradycardia, hypotension, atrioventricular blocks, hypoglycemia, bronchospasm, hyperkalemia, seizures, respiratory arrest	IV fluids, atropine; glucagon 3–10 mg IV bolus followed by infusion of 2–5 mg/h; catecholamine pressors

CNS = central nervous system; ECG = electrocardiogram; IV = intravenously; ms = milliseconds; PO = by mouth.

12
CHAPTER

Obstetric and Gynecologic Problems

PREHOSPITAL CONSIDERATIONS

▶ All women of childbearing age with a history of vaginal bleeding or abdominal pain are at risk of becoming hemodynamically unstable and require the establishment of IV access with at least one large-bore catheter.
▶ Rapid infusion of 1 to 2 liters of normal saline is required in all hemodynamically unstable women with vaginal bleeding.

In this chapter, we present the two major problems seen in the ED that are specific to women: pelvic pain and vaginal bleeding. As an emergency physician, place emphasis on recognizing conditions that can threaten a patient's life or fertility. In particular, rapidly assess the patient's hemodynamic stability and, if it is compromised, initiate resuscitative efforts while facilitating timely gynecologic consultation. Also, determine whether or not the patient is pregnant. **PEARL: Obtain β-HCG (serum beta human chorionic gonadotropin) on all women of childbearing age with**

abdominal pain or vaginal bleeding. Pelvic ultrasonography, both transabdominal and transvaginal, is an extremely helpful diagnostic tool for delineating adnexal and uterine pathology and should be used in conjunction with gynecologic consultation whenever indicated.

PELVIC PAIN

In addition to considering all the diagnostic possibilities discussed in the chapter on abdominal pain, emphasis should be placed on ruling out potentially life-threatening conditions, such as an ectopic pregnancy, a ruptured hemorrhagic ovarian cyst, and a ruptured tubo-ovarian abscess. Early recognition and treatment of an ectopic pregnancy can be life-saving and can help prevent infertility and recurrences. Always assume that a woman of child-bearing age is pregnant until proven otherwise.

History

Include the following information in the patient's history:
- Prior pregnancy, abortion, miscarriage, and live births.
- Details of associated abdominal pain (location, radiation, and aggravating and relieving factors) or gastrointestinal symptoms such as nausea, vomiting, or diarrhea.
- The temporal relation of the pain to menses and coitus.
- A detailed menstrual history, including the regularity and specific details of the last two to three menstrual periods.
- Associated urinary frequency or dysuria.
- Associated vaginal itch, discharge, bleeding, or spotting.
- Sexual practices and the use of contraception.
- History of sexually transmitted diseases.
- History of ectopic pregnancy.
- History of dizziness or lightheadedness.
- Family and personal history of bleeding disorders.
- Use of anticoagulants or antiplatelet medications.

Physical Examination
Vital Signs

Always measure orthostatic as well as supine vital signs. If the patient is unstable, rapidly establish venous access and give fluids. Notify the Ob-Gyn consultant as soon as possible. Send blood for typing and cross-match and for β-hCG, and spin a hematocrit (see the following section on laboratory tests). If patient is in shock, give O-negative blood. A rapid bedside ultrasound evaluating for the presence of free intraperitoneal fluid will help identify women requiring rapid consultation and surgical intervention.

Pelvic Examination

PEARL: Perform pelvic examination on all women of childbearing age with abdominal pain or pelvic pain without obvious cause. Inspect the external genitalia for skin lesions before you insert a vaginal speculum. Lubricants facilitate the ease of the examination, but they have a bacteriostatic effect. Therefore, if you suspect infection, use warm water as a lubricant. Note the presence of any lesions or sources of bleeding. Is the external cervical os open or closed? Is there any blood or discharge from the cervix? Are there any lesions on the cervix itself?

Next, perform a bimanual examination. Evaluate for cervical motion tenderness; patency of the cervical os; uterine size, tenderness, and consistency; and the presence of adnexal masses or tenderness.

Sexually Transmitted Diseases

Always obtain cervical cultures for gonococcal and chlamydial infection while performing the examination with a speculum. If an abnormal discharge or abnormal findings on bimanual examination is noted, also obtain a venereal disease research laboratory (VDRL) test.

Trichomonas vaginalis infection is characterized by copious, malodorous, foamy yellow-green vaginal discharge. Diagnosis is made microscopically by identification of the parasites on a wet smear (Fig. 12–1). Metronidazole 500 mg PO bid for 7 days or a single oral dose of metronidazole 2 g is used for treatment. Note, however, that metronidazole is contraindicated in pregnancy.

Candidiasis is characterized by a white, cheesy vaginal discharge, often with significant erythema and pruritus of the vulva and vagina. The spores or pseudohyphae of *Candida albicans* ("meatballs and spaghetti" appearance) can be seen on microscopy after application of 10% KOH to a smear of the discharge (Fig. 12–2). Treatment with one oral dose of fluconazole 150 mg enhances compliance.

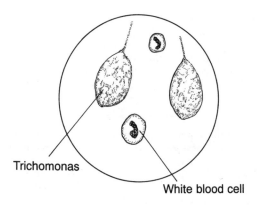

Figure 12–1. A trichomonad seen in a wet smear at high-power magnification.

Bacterial vaginosis is characterized by a thin, gray, homogenous, malodorous discharge. Pruritus is uncommon; the discharge is increased by menses and intercourse. Typically, the addition of 10% KOH to a slide containing a discharge smear produces a fishy odor. Bacterial vaginosis is caused by a variety of bacteria, such as *Gardnerella vaginalis,* and is characterized by a vaginal pH > 4.5. Diagnosis is supported by the presence of clue cells [epithelial cells

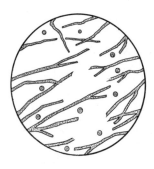

Figure 12–2. *Candida albicans* seen as spores and pseudohyphae in a KOH smear.

with bacteria adherent to their borders (Fig. 12–3)]. Treatment can be accomplished with 0.75% metronidazole vaginal gel applied twice daily for 5 days or with 2% clindamycin vaginal cream applied before bedtime for 7 days.

Laboratory Tests

In the presence of pelvic pain, the following laboratory tests are recommended: a serum β-hCG; CBC; electrolyte, glucose, BUN, and creatinine values; urinalysis; and cervical cultures. In cases of hemodynamic compromise, obtain a rapid assessment of the hematocrit by spinning a "crit." Spin a blood-filled micropipette for 60 seconds in a miniature centrifuge, and obtain the hematocrit by dividing the height of RBCs by the total height of the column. An erythrocyte sedimentation rate may be helpful when pelvic inflammatory disease (PID) is considered.

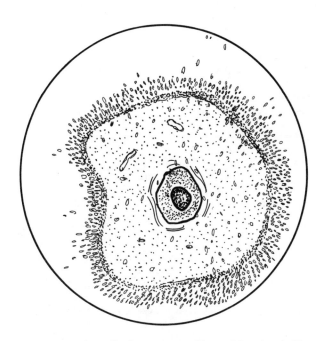

Figure 12–3. Clue cells characteristic of bacterial vaginosis. Note the epithelial cell coated with bacteria.

Specific Conditions Causing Pelvic Pain

Ectopic Pregnancy

Ectopic pregnancy occurs in 1% to 2% of all pregnancies. **PEARL: Obtain a history of risk factors for ectopic pregnancy in all women of childbearing age.** Risk factors include:

- History of PID
- History of an ectopic pregnancy
- Previous pelvic surgery
- History of tubal sterilization
- Use of an intrauterine contraceptive device
- History of induced abortions

Classically, the patient presents with a short period of amenorrhea followed by pain and abnormal bleeding. The pain usually is unilateral, but it may be diffuse and may or may not precede bleeding. Unilateral lower quadrant tenderness is common, although the patient can have a normal exam. Unilateral adnexal tenderness or a mass may be found. The uterus may be of normal size and, if enlarged, is often smaller than expected by date of pregnancy.

In about 10% of cases, the ectopic pregnancy ruptures and significant intraperitoneal bleeding occurs; the patient can present with syncope, shock, or signs of peritoneal irritation. Shoulder pain, especially in the supine position, may be due to diaphragmatic irritation from intraperitoneal bleeding. A positive pregnancy test confirms the presence of a pregnancy, either intrauterine or ectopic. If the patient is unstable, immediate surgery is required, often before the results of the pregnancy test are available.

In all cases of suspected ectopic pregnancy, IV access with two large-bore angiocatheters should be established. **PEARL: Get bedside ultrasound and an Ob-Gyn consultation as early as possible in women with hemodynamic instability to expedite diagnosis and management.** In the stable patient, pelvic ultrasound (abdominal or intravaginal) should be performed to look for an intrauterine gestational sac (which usually rules out an ectopic pregnancy) as well as adnexal masses or sacs. A gestational sac should be evident by 4 to 5 weeks, a fetal pole by 5 to 6 weeks, and fetal heart motion by 6 to 7 weeks. The result of a quantitative β-hCG test, when available, is extremely helpful. An intrauterine pregnancy should be present on intravaginal ultrasound when the β-hCG level is >1500 to 2000 mIU/L. Absence of a gestational sac on intravaginal ultrasound in a patient with a β-hCG above this discriminatory zone is highly suggestive of an ectopic pregnancy.

Knowledge of your laboratory's threshold for detecting β-hCG is crucial for appropriate interpretation. Most labs are able to detect a level > 25 mIU/L in the serum and > 50 mIU/L in the urine. Rapid administration of fluids or a dilute urine can reduce the test's sensitivity. When available, a progesterone level greater than 5 ng/mL suggests a normal intrauterine pregnancy.

If the patient is unstable, perform a culdocentesis to determine the presence of nonclotting blood. (A negative culdocentesis rules out hemoperitoneum but does not exclude the possibility of an extrauterine pregnancy.) To perform a culdocentesis, insert a vaginal speculum and grab the posterior cervical lip with a tenaculum. Insert a #18 spinal needle attached to a 10-mL syringe through the posterior fornix into the cul de sac (Fig. 12–4). To avoid uterine penetration, continuously pull back on the plunger until you get a free flow of fluid or blood, indicating entry into the peritoneal cavity. Aspiration of > 5 to 10 mL of nonclotting blood is evidence of intraperitoneal hemorrhage. A rapid bedside ultrasound can also be used to identify free intraperitoneal fluid.

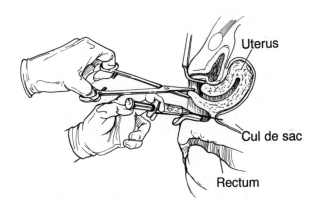

Figure 12–4. Culdocentesis. The posterior cervical lip is grasped with a tenaculum while blood is aspirated from the cul de sac.

Ovarian Torsion

Ovarian torsion can occur in the presence of ovarian or fallopian pathology. Patients present with sudden onset of unilateral pain, which may be sharp or dull, constant or intermittent. Patients usually are afebrile. Physical examination reveals unilateral lower quadrant tenderness with or without signs of peritonitis. Most patients have unilateral adnexal tenderness and a mass, as well as some cervical motion tenderness.

The differential diagnosis includes unilateral PID, acute appendicitis, and ectopic pregnancy. If you suspect ovarian torsion, seek early gynecologic consultation and perform pelvic ultrasound, preferably with color-flow Doppler imaging.

Ovarian Cysts

Ovarian cysts are very common and often are asymptomatic. Symptomatic cysts are most often secondary to rupture, torsion, infection, or bleeding. Ovarian cysts can be *functional* (follicular or corpus luteum), *benign* (dermoid, teratoma), or *malignant*. Patients with a ruptured ovarian cyst can present with a sudden onset of unilateral, sharp pelvic pain, often after exertion or coitus. On examination, patients are afebrile and may show signs of hemodynamic instability. Unilateral adnexal tenderness or a mass, together with signs of peritoneal irritation, may be present. Mittelschmerz occurs at midcycle in up to 25% of women due to rupture of a follicular cyst at the time of ovulation and manifests as unilateral pelvic pain lasting hours to several days.

Most small ovarian masses, especially if they enlarge before ovulation or menstruation, are benign. Women with an adnexal mass, however, should be reassessed by a gynecologist after their menses. All patients with signs of peritoneal irritation or hemodynamic instability must be seen urgently by a gynecologist.

Pelvic Inflammatory Disease

In PID, the pain often is bilateral and accompanied by bilateral adnexal tenderness, cervical discharge, and prominent cervical motion tenderness. Patients who are discharged should be treated with ceftriaxone 250 mg IM followed by doxycycline 100 mg PO twice daily for 10 to 14 days. PID is discussed in more detail in Chapter 14 on sexually transmitted diseases (STDs).

Endometriosis

Endometriosis is the result of the abnormal location of endometrial tissue outside of the uterus (usually in the pelvis). Classically, the patient is in her late 20s or early 30s and presents with a combination of the following symptoms: *dysmenorrhea* (pain around menses), *dyspareunia* (pain during sexual intercourse), *menstrual abnormalities*, and *infertility*. Pain is bilateral and dull and becomes progressively worse toward the end of the menstrual cycle. Bladder or bowel involvement can cause symptoms related to function of these organs. Rarely, sensitive nodules can be palpated on pelvic or rectal examination. The stable patient with presumed endometriosis should be referred to a gynecologist for consideration of hormonal therapy (danazol). Pain can be managed with NSAIDs.

VAGINAL BLEEDING

The Normal Menses

The average age of menarche is 12 years; the average age of onset of menopause is 48 years. The length of the menstrual cycle varies from 18 to 40 days. Bleeding is heaviest during the first 2 days and lasts 3 to 7 days. The average blood loss is 25 to 60 mL. The degree of blood loss can be estimated from the number of pads or tampons needed. An average tampon absorbs as much as 20 to 30 mL of blood.

Initial Assessment of Vaginal Bleeding

When a women presents with vaginal bleeding, two questions must be answered as soon as possible.

1. Is the vaginal bleeding causing hemodynamic compromise?
2. Is the patient pregnant?

Assessment of the patient's ABCs, as well as orthostatic changes in the BP and pulse, should be measured as soon as possible. If the patient has evidence of hemodynamic compromise, immediately establish IV access with two large-bore IV catheters and initiate fluid resuscitation. Blood should be sent for a blood typing and cross-match, CBC, platelets, prothrombin time (PT), partial thromboplastin time (PTT), and a serum β-hCG. Have the blood bank type and cross-match 4 U of packed red blood cells. A gynecologist should be involved as soon as possible. Hemorrhaging can be controlled by packing the vagina with sterile towels until the operating room is available.

Vaginal Bleeding in the Nonpregnant Woman

Dysfunctional bleeding, secondary to a nonovulatory cycle, is the most common cause of vaginal bleeding in women of childbearing age. This is commonly seen around menarche or menopause, but can occur at any point in the cycle; it rarely leads to hemodynamic compromise. **PEARL: Hemodynamically stable nonpregnant women with vaginal bleeding and adequate hematocrit can be discharged safely from the hospital with early follow-up by a gynecologist.** If bleeding is profuse but the patient is hemodynamically stable and has a hematocrit within normal limits, medroxyprogesterone (Provera, The Upjohn Company, Kalamazoo, MI) 10 mg PO four times daily for 10 days or conjugated estrogens tablets (Premarin, Wyeth-Ayerst Laboratories, Philadelphia, PA) 2.5 mg PO four times daily for 21 days followed by medroxyprogesterone for the last 5 days can be given in consultation with a gynecologist.

Other causes of vaginal bleeding in the nonpregnant woman include *neoplasms* and *trauma*. A thorough pelvic examination picks up many of these illnesses, which will need gynecologic follow-up. A *generalized coagulopathy* should be suspected when a patient has a personal or family history of a bleeding tendency (blood in urine or stool, bleeding from gums, or easy bruising) and is evaluated with a PT, PTT, and a platelet count. Always ask whether the patient is on any anticoagulant agents or NSAIDs. Postmenopausal bleeding always should be presumed to be caused by neoplasms until proven otherwise. In children, suspect *foreign bodies* or *sexual abuse*.

Table 12–1. DIFFERENTIATING PLACENTAL ABRUPTION FROM PLACENTA PREVIA

Parameter	Placental Abruption	Placenta Previa
Vaginal bleeding	Dark red, purple	Bright red
Pain	Severe	Absent or minimal
Uterine tenderness	Significant	Absent
Degree of shock	Out of proportion to external bleeding	Proportional to degree of external bleeding
Risk factors	Advanced maternal age and parity	Multiparity
	Maternal hypertension	Prior cesarean section
	Smoking history	

Vaginal Bleeding in Early Pregnancy

First-trimester bleeding may be due to any of the causes of vaginal bleeding in the nonpregnant woman, as well as to a spontaneous abortion, an ectopic pregnancy, or gestational trophoblastic disease.

Patients having *spontaneous abortions* present with painless vaginal bleeding sometimes followed by crampy abdominal pain; bleeding preceded by pain is more characteristic of ectopic pregnancy. Perform an abdominal examination to assess for tenderness or signs of peritoneal irritation. On the pelvic examination, note whether the external cervical os is open or closed and whether any clots or fetal tissue are evident. Microscopic evaluation of any passed tissue (in saline suspension) may show feathery-appearing chorionic villi.

Anti-D immune globulin (RhoGAM, Ortho Diagnostic Systems, a Johnson & Johnson Co., Raritan, NJ) 300 μg IM should be considered if the patient is Rh-negative; this protects against a fetal–maternal hemorrhage of up to 30 mL. Ob-Gyn consultation should be obtained in all cases of abortion, whether threatened, incomplete, or complete. The patient often requires a dilation and curettage.

Vaginal Bleeding in Later Pregnancy

Vaginal bleeding during the third trimester is usually caused by either *placental abruption* or *placenta previa*. As always, assess the ABCs and determine the hemodynamic stability of the patient. Two large-bore IV catheters should be established, and blood should be sent for typing and cross-match, CBC, platelets, PT, PTT, fibrinogen, and fibrin split products [the latter to assess for disseminated intravascular coagulation (DIC) associated with placental abruption].

In the presence of placenta previa, a pelvic examination can cause catastrophic bleeding. **PEARL: Avoid manual pelvic examinations in patients with vaginal bleeding during late pregnancy.** Assessment for fetal heart tones should be made with a portable Doppler. Once the patient is stable, she should be transferred to the delivery suite for further evaluation and management. Emergency pelvic ultrasound is extremely helpful in excluding a placenta previa. Table 12–1 distinguishes placental abruption from placenta previa.

13

Common Pediatric Problems

PREHOSPITAL CONSIDERATIONS

▶ Hypoxia is the pathway to decompensation in children.
▶ Always use 100% oxygen for any signs of respiratory distress, especially in newborns.
▶ Children are extremely anxious about the ambulance ride. Reassure and talk with the patient.

This chapter covers selected topics in emergency pediatrics and includes some useful tricks and methods that will help you in dealing with the sick child. The cliché bears repeating: "Children are not just little adults." Some techniques, such as intubation, are somewhat different in children. Vital signs differ by age. This chapter also includes sections on two specific pediatric problem areas: the airway and fever. The last section of the chapter covers the topic of sedation. **PEARL: Consider hypoglycemia in all unstable or toxic children. Do a rapid bedside test early.**

GENERAL CONSIDERATIONS

In most cases, you'll have time to calculate drug dosages based on the child's weight. **PEARL: Medications must always**

be age- and weight-appropriate. When this is not possible, as in a code, several approximation methods are useful. The Broselow tape is a measuring device that every ED should have. **PEARL: Use of the Broselow tape will aid in the knowledge of equipment sizes and drug dosages.** To use it, merely measure the child's length with it, and then read off the proper drug doses and equipment sizes. When this tape is not available, you will have to estimate the weight: a 1-year-old infant weighs approximately 10 kg and a 5-year-old child approximately 20 kg. For children between the ages of 1 and 8 years, a useful formula is as follows:

$$\text{Weight (kg)} = (\text{age} \times 2) + 8$$

Practice estimating weights with all the children you see.

Normal vital signs do vary by age. Table 13–1 is a rough guide. The following is a useful formula for estimating minimum systolic BP.

$$\text{Minimum systolic BP} = 70 + (\text{age} \times 2)$$

Children tend to compensate well for illnesses until the moment of collapse. An adult who loses 30% of blood volume will be hypotensive, but a child with similar losses would show tachycardia but probably a preserved BP until the time he or she arrests. In other words, children may appear deceptively well before decompensating. The lesson is that you must pay attention to the child's clinical appearance. **PEARL: In children, even more than in adults, what the patient "looks like" is the best indicator of clinical status.** This judgment comes only with experience; try to develop

Table 13–1. NORMAL VITAL SIGNS BY AGE

Age	Respirations*	Pulse†	Systolic BP (mm Hg)
Newborn	40	140–160	60
3–6 months	30–40	120–140	80
1 year	20–30	110–130	90–100
5 years	20	100–110	100
8 years	12–20	90–100	105

*In breaths per minute.
†In beats per minute.
BP = blood pressure.

it while you are in the ED. Use the level of the child's playfulness in the ED as an indicator. In children, it often is helpful to assess capillary refill. Cool or clammy extremities as well as a prolonged capillary refill suggest shock.

Pediatric codes tend to frighten and even "paralyze" novice clinicians. People tend to focus on one task, such as attempting IV access, to the exclusion of taking care of the patient. Therefore, in addition to the ABCs, we offer you the "Seven Points of Light" that should be done for every pediatric code (note that none of them is IV access):

1. Oxygen.
2. History: Assign someone to gather this information from the persons who brought the child in.
3. Physical examination: Look for signs of trauma or petechial rash (possible sepsis).
4. Temperature: measured rectally. Look for hypothermia and fever.
5. Heel-stick blood: for spun hematocrit.
6. Heel-stick blood: for glucose chemstrip.
7. Cardiac monitor leads.

You should also, of course, intubate the patient and obtain venous or intraosseous access.

Fluid management for children in the emergency setting is simpler than longer-term calculations. In general, any dehydrated child should receive a bolus of normal saline of 20 mL/kg IV. Repeat until vital signs stabilize. Note that if the child's volume loss is due to bleeding, give PRBCs at 10 mL/kg after the second fluid bolus. The degree of dehydration (*not* blood volume loss) can be estimated based on clinical signs. A child with mild (5%) dehydration has dry mucous membranes but otherwise appears normal. At a moderate (10%) level, the child is also tachycardic, with sunken eyeballs and fontanel, and may be hypotensive. Severe (15%) dehydration is accompanied by additional symptoms of poor skin turgor, an altered sensorium, metabolic acidosis, poor capillary refill, and frank hypotension.

Once the patient is stable, calculate maintenance fluid requirements. An easy formula is as follows:

4 mL/kg per hour for the first 10 kg of weight
2 mL/kg per hour for the next 10 kg
1 mL/kg per hour for every kilogram thereafter

For example, a 23-kg child requires maintenance fluid as follows:

$$(4 \times 10) + (2 \times 10) + (1 \times 3) = 63 \text{ mL/hour}$$

The usual fluid for children under 10 kg is D_5W in 0.25 NS (Isolyte P with 5% Dextrose, American McGaw, Santa Ana, CA). For children over 10 kg, use $D_5W/0.45$ NS. In the setting of dehydration, the deficit also needs to be replaced; for hypotonic (hyponatremic) and isotonic dehydration, NS usually is given over a 24-hour period. For hypertonic (hypernatremic) dehydration, replacement fluid (usually D_5W) must be given over 48 hours to avoid cerebral edema. Note that the child should be receiving maintenance fluid as well during this period.

Some useful information on pediatric immunizations and oral drug dosing can be found in Tables 13–2 and 13–3.

THE PEDIATRIC AIRWAY

Adults tend to die cardiac deaths; children tend to die respiratory deaths. **PEARL: The common pathway to cardiopulmonary collapse in most children is respiratory failure and/or shock.**

Supporting a child's respiratory status often is the deciding factor in saving his or her life. Intubation of a child—essentially the same procedure as in an adult—has

Table 13–2. PEDIATRIC IMMUNIZATION SCHEDULE

Age	Immunizations
Birth	HBV
2 months	DTP, HbCV, OPV, HBV
4 months	DTP, HbCV, OPV
6 months	DTP, HbCV, HBV
15 months	MMR, HbCV
15–18 months	DTP, OPV
4–6 years	DTP, OPV
4–12 years	MMR
14–16 years	Td

DTP = diphtheria, tetanus, and pertussis vaccine; HbCV = *Haemophilus influenzae* conjugate vaccine; HBV = hepatitis B vaccine; MMR = measles, mumps, and rubella vaccine; OPV = oral polio vaccine; Td = tetanus and diphtheria adult formulation vaccine.

Table 13–3. COMMON PEDIATRIC ORAL DRUG DOSES

Generic Name (Brand Name)	Formulation	Dose
Acetaminophen (Tylenol)	80 mg/0.8 mL 160 mg/5 mL 80-mg chewtab	15 mg/kg q 4 hours
Ibuprofen (Pediaprofen)	100 mg/5 mL	10 mg/kg q 6 hours
Albuterol (Proventil)	2 mg/5 mL	2–5 years: 0.1 mg/kg tid 6–11 years: 2 mg tid 12+ years: 2 mg tid–qid
Prednisone (Pediapred)	5 or 25 mg/5 mL	2 mg/kg/day
Amoxicillin (Amoxil)	125 mg/5 mL 250 mg/5 mL	10 mg/kg tid
Penicillin V potassium (Pen Vee K)	125 mg/5 mL 250 mg/5 mL	10 mg/kg qid
Cephalexin (Keflex)	125 mg/5 mL 250 mg/5 mL	10 mg/kg qid
Trimethoprim-sulfamethoxazole (Bactrim, Septra)	TMP 40 mg and SMX 200 mg/5 mL	Based on TMP as TMP 4 mg/kg bid
Erythromycin-sulfamethoxazole (Pediazole)	200 mg EM and 600 mg SMX/5 mL	By weight: 8 kg: 2.5 mL qid 16 kg: 5 mL qid 24 kg: 7.5 mL qid >45 kg: 10 mL qid
Clarithromycin (Biaxin)	125–250 mg/5 mL	7.5 mg/kg bid
Azithromycin (Zithromax)	100–200 mg/5 mL	10 mg/kg single dose, followed by 5 mg daily for 4 more days

EM = erythromycin; SMX = sulfamethoxazole; TMP = trimethoprim.

some quirks. Tube size depends on the age of the child; use the following formula to estimate it.

$$\text{Tube size (mm)} = 4 + \frac{\text{child's age}}{4}$$

Children's tubes (up to size 6, about age 5) are uncuffed, because, unlike in an adult, the tightest area of the airway is subglottic. A straight (Miller) laryngoscope blade may be easier to use because a child's epiglottis is longer, floppier, and more anterior than an adult's. Also, because of a child's smaller size, it's easier to intubate the right main-stem bronchus, so be wary of this and try to avoid passing the tube too deep. The distance from the teeth to the carina can be estimated by the following formula.

$$\text{Distance (cm)} = 12 + \frac{\text{child's age}}{2}$$

Try not to hyperextend the child's neck because this brings the larynx even more anterior and complicates the intubation. At the end of the endotracheal tube are two black stripes. The first stripe should be passed beyond the vocal cords; leave the second stripe above the cords, which will ensure that the tube is always in place. The hardest part of intubation is ensuring that the tube stays in place—holding it and securing it with tape is essential! If you're having difficulty with intubation, consider doing a digital intubation after visualizing or palpating the epiglottis.

Epiglottitis

Once believed to be almost exclusively a disease of children, it is seen in all age groups. Since the Hib vaccine has had widespread use, the number of childhood epiglottitis cases has dropped significantly. *Staphylococcus aureus, Streptococcus pneumoniae,* and other bacteria can still be responsible for acute epiglottis in children as well as in adults. Because of the small size of a child's airway, a disease such as epiglottitis can be rapidly life-threatening. Typically, a child with this infectious disorder presents with a high fever, "toxic" (i.e., very sick) appearance, drooling, and sitting up on both arms (the "tripod" position). The voice is often muffled. **PEARL: When you suspect epiglottitis, do not agitate the child or put anything in his or her mouth, because this can cause acute airway obstruction by provoking laryngospasm.** Immediately notify the operating room, anesthesiologist, and ENT or pediatric surgeon. Often, the next step is to take the patient immediately to the operating room for a controlled intubation. Starting an IV is best deferred until the airway is secured, again because of possibly causing a complete airway obstruction. If the child's airway becomes blocked, all attempts at intubation must be done in the ED. If you have a low suspicion for epiglottitis and the child is stable, take a lateral neck x-ray of the soft tissues; epiglottitis is evidenced by a "thumbprint" (i.e., swollen) epiglottis and the loss of the vallecular space (vallecula sign). Children who are ill appearing without having evidence of epiglottitis may have bacterial tracheitis, which can be serious and would require admission, especially for pulmonary toilet, which almost always requires intubation. Making a diagnosis in older children may be difficult. The complaint of a severe sore throat without any visual evidence of pharyngitis may be the only clue to the diagnosis. Direct visualization with a flexible laryngoscopy can be necessary. Epiglottis can also be present with an acute uvulitis.

Croup

Croup, another common pediatric airway problem, is an infectious disease—laryngotracheobronchitis caused by parainfluenza virus. In general, croup is not life-threatening and can be treated easily with humidified oxygen and occasionally, corticosteroids (dexamethasone 0.6 mg/kg IM). The main difficulty is in distinguishing it from epiglottitis or other serious upper airway infections. This can be accomplished on clinical grounds, as shown in Table 13–4. Children should be immediately treated with humidified oxygen in the arms of the parent. Severe respiratory distress can be treated with nebulized racemic epinephrine 0.5 mL of the 2.25% solution in 3 mL of saline. Previously feared rebound phenomenon seems uncommon, although some patients return to their baseline after the drug wears off and, therefore, should be observed 4 to 6 hours before discharge. Severe respiratory distress or resting stridor is an indication for corticosteroids.

Asthma

Asthma is an extremely common pediatric problem consisting of reversible bronchospasm, most often caused by

Table 13–4. CROUP VERSUS EPIGLOTTITIS

	Croup	Epiglottitis
Age	6 months to 5 years; peak 2 years	3 to 6 years
Gender	M > F, 2:1	M = F
Season	Fall and winter	Variable
Etiology	Viral, usually parainfluenza	Bacterial, usually *H. influenzae* B
Prodrome	Upper respiratory infection	Usually none
Onset	Gradual	Rapid
Fever	Low-grade	High
Toxic?	No	Yes
Sore throat?	Variable	Yes
Voice	Hoarse	Muffled
Drooling?	No	Yes
Cough	Barking, "croupy"	No
Position	Variable	Prefers sitting or "tripod" position
WBC count*	Normal	High
Blood culture*	Negative	Positive
Lateral neck x-ray	"Steeple sign"	"Thumbprint" epiglottis

*Caution: In suspected epiglottitis, do not draw blood or do anything to agitate the patient until the ENT and anesthesia teams are ready to manage the patient's airway (usually in the operating room.)
ENT = ear, nose, and throat; F = female; M = male; WBC = white blood cell.

allergies or concurrent infection. The mainstay of management is nebulized β-adrenergic agonists such as albuterol or metaproterenol. The usual dose of albuterol is 2.5 mg in 2 mL of saline nebulized every 20 minutes until the attack is broken. Many studies show that this drug also can be given continuously for 1 hour with relatively few side effects. Ipratropiun bromide (Atrovent), when used in combination with albuterol, has additional beneficial effects. This should be added to the first dose of albuterol during the ED management of the patient. To document improvement, we like to follow peak flow readings in children old enough to cooperate; this is especially useful in patients with known baseline peak flow values. Pulse oximetry also is helpful; it can warn of hypoxia, which indicates the need for admission.

Our standard method of treatment is to give the child three nebulizer treatments and then reassess. If the child still has slight wheezing or slightly reduced peak flow but otherwise seems well, we discharge the child on β-agonists and corticosteroids, such as prednisone 2 mg/kg per day. If the child is completely back to normal, we may forgo the corticosteroids. Indications for chest x-ray include:

- A first episode of wheezing
- Fever
- Asymmetric lung exam
- Chest pain
- Hypoxia
- An intractable attack (requiring more than three nebulizer treatments)
- Hospital admission

Indications for hospital admission include:

- Hypoxia (pulse oximeter < 94%)
- Intractable attack
- Concurrent infection
- Progressive fatigue
- Poor parental compliance and follow-up
- History of respiratory failure and previous intubations

In the most severe attacks, when patients are not responding to standard therapy, use systemic epinephrine (0.01 mg/kg up to 0.3 mg SC every 20 minutes × 3 doses), parenteral terbutaline (0.01 mL up to 0.25 mL/dose every 20 minutes SC), methylprednisolone (1 to 2 mg/kg/dose), magnesium sulfate, or ketamine. Theophylline has not been shown to augment bronchodilatation in the setting of maximal β-adrenergic treatment. Patients in respiratory failure must be intubated.

NEONATAL ILLNESSES

Respiratory Distress

Apnea, common in neonates, is the cessation of breathing for more than 20 seconds or with symptoms of bradycardia, cyanosis, or mental status change. These patients need to be admitted to the hospital and observed closely with electronic apnea monitoring. Patients need to be ruled out for sepsis, hypoglycemia, hypocalcemia, hypoxia, GI reflux, seizures, and hypothermia.

Bronchopulmonary dysplasia (BPD) is a common disorder in newborns who have survived the neonatal intensive care unit (NICU). Many of these infants were premature and suffer from hyaline membrane disease and may be on home O_2. The emergency physician needs to deal with the infant who decompensates and is rarely concerned with making the initial diagnosis. These patients are usually hypoxic and retain CO_2; often, their decompensation is associated with respiratory syncytial virus (RSV) infections. A chest x-ray is necessary to rule out concomitant pneumonia or atelectasis. Patients with BPD should be treated with aggressive oxygen therapy, and the wheezing can be treated with nebulized albuterol (2.5 to 5.0 mg in 2.5-mL saline solution). They should have RSV testing by nasopharyngeal swabs so that appropriate isolation can be done in the hospital. Children with underlying cardiac or lung pathology, immunodeficiency, or congenital anomalies are at greatest risk for death secondary to respiratory failure. **PEARL: In the newborn, resuscitation should focus on stimulation, oxygenation, warming, assisted ventilation, and occasionally, chest compressions. Medications are rarely necessary.**

Cyanosis

Cyanosis is a physical *sign* characterized by a bluish discoloration of the skin and mucous membranes. It is evident when at least 5 g of reduced hemoglobin is present in 100 mL of capillary blood. This increased amount of reduced hemoglobin can be due to many different conditions, including cardiac, pulmonary, congenital, trauma, or blood disorders. Peripheral cyanosis is a bluish discoloration resulting from slowing of the blood flow to an area in which there is an increased extraction of oxygen from normal arterial blood. This is seen in children with sepsis and shock states and in newborns with temperature changes. It is not uncommon for NICU graduates to have various congenital heart diseases that would present in the ED with cyanosis. Congenital heart disease often presents as CHF.

CHF in the newborn can be difficult to diagnos. The most common complaint is that the child is not feeding well or may have some respiratory distress. Physical examination may demonstrate mottled skin, grunting, nasal flaring, rales on auscultation of the chest, or an enlarged liver. Chest x-ray is helpful, often showing an enlarged heart and increased pulmonary vascular markings. Treatment consists of oxygen and furosemide (1 mg/kg IV). Digoxin therapy can be used in chronic cases of heart failure in neonates. Consultation with a pediatric cardiologist should be done in the ED. In tetralogy of Fallot, cyanosis is caused by decreased blood flow to the pulmonary bed and a right-to-left shunt and may be seen with CHF or hypercyanotic spells. These patients require high-flow oxygen and should be put into a squatting position to decrease right blood flow. All these patients with congenital heart disorders require treatment that goes beyond the emergency medicine practice, and early consultation with a pediatric cardiologist is strongly advised.

Jaundice

Jaundice is one of the most common neonatal problems that only occasionally causes any true emergency. Physiologic jaundice is commonly seen in neonates because of a decrease in normal liver enzymes, which leads to an elevated indirect bilirubin.

The causes of nonphysiologic jaundice include:
- Sepsis
- Polycythemia
- Inborn errors of metabolism
- Fetal-maternal blood group incompatibility
- Hypothyroidism
- Breast milk jaundice
- Direct hyperbilirubinemia

Physiologic jaundice is a diagnosis of exclusion. Testing

to rule out the above conditions is necessary. The total bilirubin level is usually < 13 mg/dL. Sepsis should be ruled out based on H&P, CBC, urinalysis, chest x-ray, and cultures. Hemolytic processes, which will demonstrate an abnormal CBC with an elevated reticulocyte count, should also be excluded.

FEVER AND INFECTIOUS DISEASES

Although the most common cause of fever is a benign viral infection, a child younger than 2 years with fever can have such serious illnesses as meningitis or bacteremia without any obvious findings. Workup of fever in a child, therefore, depends on the child's age. Here, we will discuss the management of a child who has fever *without* a known source. If a focus of infection is found, treat the child as appropriate for that infection. The approaches discussed as follows have been suggested by a panel of pediatricians and emergency physicians who met to develop the American College of Emergency Physicians' guidelines and are summarized in Figures 13–1 and 13–2.

Newborn

In the newborn and infants up to 4 weeks of age, any fever warrants a full sepsis workup—blood culture, catheterized

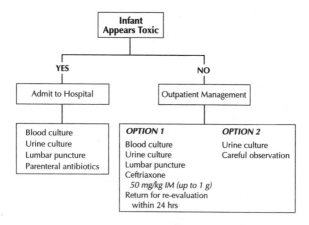

Figure 13–1. Management of a previously healthy low-risk infant aged 28 to 90 days old, with a fever without a source.

or suprapubic urine culture, lumbar puncture (LP), and chest x-ray. The child should then be started on IV antibiotics, usually ampicillin 50 mg/kg IV every 8 hours, and gentamicin 1.5 mg/kg IV every 8 hours, or cefotaxime 200 mg/kg per day IV in three divided doses. The child should be hospitalized until culture results come back.

Infant 28 to 90 Days Old

Children between 28 and 90 days of age should be classified as *low risk* or *high risk*. A child is considered low risk if he or she meets *all* of the following criteria:

- Previously healthy
- Appears nontoxic
- No focal bacterial infection except otitis media
- Good social situation with reliable follow-up
- WBC count between 5000 and 15,000/mL with fewer than 1500 band forms
- Less than 5 WBC/high-power field on urinalysis (catheterized or suprapubic sample)
- Less than 5 WBC/high-power field in stool, if diarrhea present

The workup of a febrile infant requires blood drawing for the CBC, so it is usually a good idea to draw blood for a culture at the same time in case you decide to order one. This saves the child another needle stick. High-risk children are pan-cultured as above and admitted to the hospital. For the low-risk child, there are two generally accepted options (see Fig. 13–1). The one you use depends on your local protocols or clinical experience:

- Option 1: Send a urine culture to the lab and discharge the child with close follow-up [i.e., to be seen again in the ED or by the primary pediatrician within 12 to 24 hours (call the pediatrician to let him or her know)]. Warn the caregiver to bring the child back if *any* worsening occurs, and prescribe acetaminophen 15 mg/kg given orally or rectally every 4 hours for fever.
- Option 2: Send a blood culture *and* perform an LP for CSF cell count and culture; then give the child ceftriaxone 50 mg/kg IM. This provides 24 hours of IV-equivalent antibiotic coverage. This child also *must* be seen again in 24 hours to receive another dose of ceftriaxone. If the blood and CSF cultures are negative at 48 hours, antibiotics then can be discontinued.

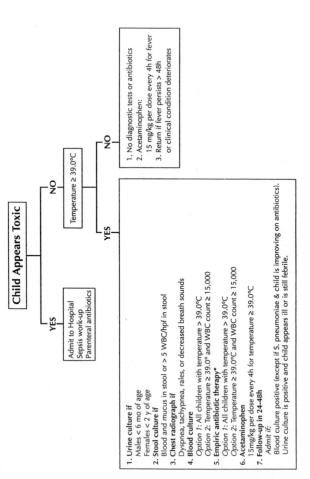

Child Appears Toxic

YES

Admit to Hospital
Sepsis work-up
Parenteral antibiotics

NO

Temperature ≥ 39.0°C

NO

1. No diagnostic tests or antibiotics
2. Acetaminophen:
   15 mg/kg per dose every 4h for fever
3. Return if fever persists > 48h
   or clinical condition deteriorates

YES

1. **Urine culture** if
   Males < 6 mo of age
   Females < 2 y of age
2. **Stool culture** if
   Blood and mucus in stool or > 5 WBC/hpf in stool
3. **Chest radiograph** if
   Dyspnea, tachypnea, rales, or decreased breath sounds
4. **Blood culture**
   Option 1: All children with temperature > 39.0°C
   Option 2: Temperature ≥ 39.0° and WBC count ≥ 15,000
5. **Empiric antibiotic therapy***
   Option 1: All children with temperature > 39.0°C
   Option 2: Temperature ≥ 39.0°C and WBC count ≥ 15,000
6. **Acetaminophen**
   15mg/kg per dose every 4h for temperature ≥ 39.0°C
7. **Follow-up** in 24–48h
       Admit if:
       Blood culture positive (except if S. pneumoniae & child is improving on antibiotics).
       Urine culture is positive and child appears ill or is still febrile.

Figure 13–2. Management of a previously healthy child aged 3 to 24 months old, with a fever without a source

Children 12 Weeks to 2 Years

For children with fever who are between 12 weeks and 2 years of age, discharge and close follow-up are acceptable if—and only if—the child appears clinically well (see Fig. 13–2). Some clinicians send off blood cultures as a screen for bacteremia, planning on calling the patient back if the cultures are positive. The argument has been made that a WBC count of 15,000/mL or higher is predictive of bacteremia and should be used as an indication for admission for administration of IV antibiotics. Unfortunately, a WBC count this high may predict bacteremia, but it predicts only pneumococcal bacteremia. Children who have this infection, but look well, usually do well regardless of antibiotics.

Children with the far more serious *Haemophilus influenzae* bacteremia, who *do* need IV antibiotics, often have normal WBC counts. **PEARL: Therefore, do not routinely rely solely on WBC lab value for admission decisions.** We do recommend that all children up to 2 years have a urine sample cultured for possible urinary tract infection, since such an infection can result in severe kidney damage if untreated.

Children Over 2 or 3 Years

Children older than 2 or 3 years who have a fever (rectal temperature > 38°C) can be evaluated as you would any other patient. Many times, these children can tell you what hurts, and they develop the characteristic physical findings of specific infectious illnesses. Again, the single most important indicator of serious illness is how the child looks and interacts with his or her surroundings. A very common focal infection of young children is *otitis media;* thus, always examine the ears of any child you see. This disease is usually caused by a pneumococcus or by *H. influenzae* and treated with amoxicillin; if it has persisted despite this therapy, treatment with antibiotics, such as trimethoprim/sulfamethoxazole, cephalosporins, or macrolides, is warranted. Treatment for otitis media is continued for 10 days. The dosages of oral antibiotics are summarized in Table 13–3. **PEARL: In children with otitis media who cannot or will not tolerate oral antibiotic, treat with a single dose of ceftriaxone 50 mg/kg IM.**

Specific Conditions

A few words should be said about *meningitis.* In children, as in adults, the most common cause of meningitis is viral. Bacterial meningitis, however, is rightfully feared because of its high morbidity and mortality. Whenever you suspect meningitis, expedite the performance of the LP and administer IV antibiotics (cefotaxime 50 mg/kg or ceftriaxone 75 mg/kg) as soon as possible. In fact, if waiting for an LP will significantly delay therapy, draw blood cultures and give the antibiotics. The CSF Gram's stain still will be accurate, and the blood cultures may very well grow out the offending organism. Also, immune electrophoresis for bacterial antigens will be positive despite any antibiotic use. Corticosteroid therapy has been shown to reduce complications (especially auditory) in *H. influenzae* meningitis and often is used for all cases of suspected bacterial meningitis. The usual initial dose is dexamethasone 0.15 mg/kg IV simultaneously with or even slightly before the first dose of antibiotics. If possible, discuss the use of steroids with the admitting pediatrician.

Sore throat is another common infectious complaint. Be aware that only streptococcal infection requires treatment with antibiotics (usually penicillin for 10 days), and then only to prevent rheumatic fever. In many cases, this diagnosis requires culture, which takes 1 to 2 days. Some physicians wait for culture results, and others treat presumptively. In general, your choice depends on how certain you are that a follow-up appointment will be kept. Local customs or parental wishes often prevail. Although a positive rapid strep test result warrants antibiotics, a negative test should be followed by a throat culture.

Febrile seizures can be extremely frightening, but usually do not indicate meningitis or other serious disease. The mainstay of therapy is cooling, usually with antipyretics (e.g., acetaminophen and/or ibuprofen) or tepid baths. An LP to exclude meningitis in well-appearing children is usually not necessary. See Figure 13–3 for a summary of febrile seizure management.

A common question that parents have is, "Do I need to keep him home from school?" The answer is that an infectious child should be kept isolated from others until the period of infectivity has passed. Table 13–5 summarizes isolation recommendations for some common and uncommon diseases to help you in giving parents advice.

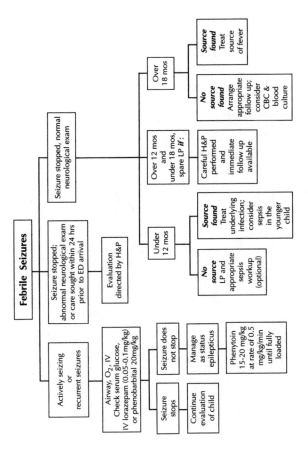

Figure 13-3. Approach to febrile seizures.

Table 13–5. PERIOD OF INFECTIVITY OF SELECTED DISEASES

Disease	Infectivity	Isolation
Chickenpox	From 1–2 days before rash appears to when all lesions are crusted (5–6 days)	From those who never had the disease, or who are immunocompromised, until all lesions crusted
Hepatitis A	1–3 weeks	Enteric precautions until asymptomatic and LFTs normal
Measles	1–2 days before rash appears until 4 days after rash appears	Respiratory isolation
Scarlet fever	Until 1–2 days of therapy complete	Until 24 hours after therapy started
Streptococcal pharyngitis	Until 1–2 days of therapy complete	Until 24 hours after therapy started

LFTs = liver function tests.

PEDIATRIC SEDATION

The ideal sedative would be painless to administer, have a rapid onset of action, have no side effects or risks, and wear off as soon as no longer needed. Of course, no real drug meets all of these criteria. Because of the inconvenience and risks of sedation, many painful and frightening procedures are performed on children using "brutane" (i.e., physical force) to accomplish. Often, if you take the time to create a comfortable setting and reassure and distract the child, less force will be needed. In addition, we believe that if properly administered and monitored, and if used in the appropriate settings (i.e., in longer and more complex procedures), sedative drugs can be used safely to minimize a child's distress in most cases. Once a child has been sedated, he or she *must* be monitored until awake. Do not discharge any child until the sedative has worn off. A child sent home sedated is an invitation to disaster.

The most effective method of sedation is to use titratable IV agents such as midazolam 0.05 to 0.10 mg/kg IV and fentanyl 1 μg/kg IV. These doses are to be repeated every 5 to 10 minutes until sedation occurs. This requires the constant attendance at the bedside of a physician and nurse skilled in pediatric resuscitation, continuous cardiac and pulse oximetry monitoring, and the availability of pediatric resuscitation equipment. Therefore, this method can be used only rarely in a busy ED, although it is often the best method for orthopedic procedures or complex suturing.

Ketamine 4 mg/kg IM or 1 mg/kg IV is a useful sedative because it does not abolish the gag reflex, and the airway thus remains relatively protected. It does produce increased secretions and should be preceded by atropine 0.01 mg/kg IV to reduce salivation. Ketamine produces dissociative amnesia in which the child appears awake but won't react to stimuli. The child receiving ketamine requires the same care and precautions as with midazolam/fentanyl sedation. To avoid "reemergence nightmares," some physicians give midazolam 0.025 mg/kg IV with the ketamine. Avoid ketamine in patients with upper airway disease, head trauma, globe injuries, or a psychiatric history. Ketamine should also be avoided if there is any chance of blood or other secretions dripping into the oropharynx.

For sedation for CT scans or other radiologic studies, we usually use secobarbital or pentobarbital 4 to 6 mg/kg IM. If the first dose does not produce adequate sedation, half of that amount can be repeated once, approximately 30 minutes after the first dose. These drugs induce 45 to 60 minutes of sedation and usually do not cause significant respiratory depression at these doses. Nevertheless, pediatric patients receiving these doses should be monitored continuously by pulse oximetry until the sedation wears off. Oral midazolam 0.1 mg/kg can also be used.

We do not recommend DPT, a combination of meperidine, promethazine, and chlorpromazine. It induces very deep and prolonged sedation and can cause dystonic reactions. Chloral hydrate is an unreliable agent, particularly in children older than 3 years; it can cause cardiac toxicity

Table 13–6. INITIAL ANTIBIOTIC THERAPY (FIRST DOSE) FOR POSSIBLE SEPSIS

Patient Characteristics	Drug	Dose (mg/kg)
Neonate (< 1 month)	Ampicillin and cefotaxime	50 50
1 month–adolescent	Cefotaxime or ceftriaxone	50 50–100
Immunocompromised	Nafcillin and ceftazidime	50 30–50
Indwelling central line	Vancomycin and ceftazidime	10–15 30–50

Table 13–7. PEDIATRIC RESUSCITATION MODALITIES

Modality	Dose/Administration and Route
Epinephrine	0.01 mg/kg; IV, ET, IO
Atropine	0.02 mg/kg; IV, ET, IO (minimum 0.1 mg/dose)
Lidocaine	1 mg/kg; IV, ET, IO to maximum of 3 mg/kg
Defibrillation	2–4 J/kg; start at 2 J/kg; double with each shock to 4 J/kg maximum
Crystalloid	20 mL/kg; IV, IO (may repeat to a total of three boluses)

ET = endotracheal tube; IO = intraosseous; IV = intravenous.

in some children even at normal doses. Regardless of the type of sedation chosen, be prepared for complications. Place all patients on a cardiac monitor and closely observe pulse oximetry.

Tables 13–6 and 13–7 provide additional information that you will find useful when providing pediatric care.

14

CHAPTER

Common Infections

PREHOSPITAL CONSIDERATIONS

▶ Patients with infections can become unstable if they develop septic shock.
▶ Unstable patients require rapid establishment of IV access and fluid resuscitation.
▶ Supplemental oxygen and active airway management may be required, particularly with respiratory infections.

Despite the abundance of antibiotics today, infectious diseases are still common and often serious illnesses. In this chapter, we briefly review several of the more common infections encountered in the ED, covering the diagnostic workup, indications for referral or admission, and the initial antibiotic choices involved in outpatient management.

Whenever indicated, obtain appropriate microbiologic specimens before you initiate therapy. The initial choice of antibiotics should be based on the most commonly infecting organisms and their local patterns of antimicrobial susceptibilities. **PEARL: Consider admitting any patient with significant underlying disease that presents with acute infection.**

URINARY TRACT INFECTIONS

In women with classic symptoms of urinary tract infection (UTI), such as dysuria and urinary frequency, a positive leukocyte esterase and/or nitrates on urine dipstick correlates highly with infection and justifies giving a course of antibiotics. In other patients, a urinalysis should be obtained. Rarely is urine culture necessary in such women. The presence of > 5 WBC per high-power field and/or bacteriuria in an unspun specimen are evidence of UTI (Fig. 14–1).

In men with symptoms of UTI, perform a rectal exam. (Avoid vigorous prostatic massage, which can cause bacteremia.) Tenderness or bogginess over the prostate gland suggests prostatitis.

A urine culture should be obtained in the following cases:
- All men and all children with UTI
- Patients with recurrent or persistent infections
- Patients with urosepsis or severe toxicity
- When the patient will be referred to a specialist

Patients should be referred to a urologist for further workup if they are:
- Young children
- Men
- Have pyelonephritis

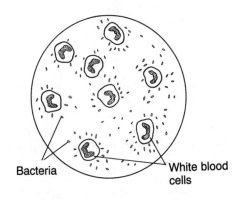

Figure 14–1. Typical microscopic findings in a urinary tract infection.

- Women with frequent infections

In the past, much emphasis was put on differentiating upper UTIs (pyelonephritis) from lower UTIs. Today, this distinction is less important in the ED because more patients with pyelonephritis are being managed as outpatients. Indications for admitting a patient with UTI include:

- Vomiting and dehydration unresponsive to oral rehydration
- Severe toxicity or sepsis
- Severe underlying diseases or immunocompromise (e.g., diabetes, steroids, or chemotherapy)
- Pregnant women with pyelonephritis (order a pregnancy test in all women of childbearing age)
- Anatomic abnormalities of the urinary tract
- Fever and costovertebral angle tenderness in patients older than 50 years

Outpatient Management

Because the most common infecting organism is *Escherichia coli* and in most areas roughly 30% of *E. coli* are resistant to ampicillin, we prefer an initial regimen of trimethoprim-sulfamethoxazole double-strength twice daily for 7 to 10 days. Alternatives include one of the fluoroquinolone regimens (e.g., ciprofloxacin 500 mg bid) and nitrofurantoin. Women with uncomplicated UTIs can be treated with a 3-day course of antibiotics if good follow-up is ensured. The acute urethral syndrome (pyuria without bacteriuria) should be treated with doxycycline, sulfamethasoxazole (Bactrim), or a fluoroquinolone with activity against *Chlamydia trachomatis* such as ofloxacin. Uncomplicated pyelonephritis should be treated for 2 weeks with Bactrim or a fluoroquinolone, or in pregnant women, a cephalosporin.

COMMUNITY-ACQUIRED PNEUMONIAS

Assessment

Most community-acquired pneumonias in the immunocompetent population are due to pneumococci, mycoplasma, or viruses. Often, the diagnosis is made based on clinical impression alone (e.g., fever, chills, productive cough, localized evidence of consolidation). Indications for a chest x-ray include:

- A low pulse oximetry reading
- Tachypnea or retractions
- Unclear diagnosis
- HIV infection
- The presence of rales (to exclude consolidation or effusion)

With the growing availability of pulse oximetry in most EDs, all patients with a diagnosis of pneumonia should have oximetry readings taken.

Disposition

Indications for admission include:

- Severe toxicity or sepsis
- Recurrent vomiting and dehydration
- Hypoxia requiring supplemental O_2 to maintain an O_2 saturation > 90% or a Po_2 > 70
- Severe underlying disease or immunocompromise (e.g., diabetes, chronic obstructive pulmonary disease, congestive heart failure, or malignancy)
- Poor social support and lack of good medical follow-up
- Extremes of age (infants and elderly)
- Failure of a trial of outpatient management
- Multilobar pneumonia or a pleural effusion
- High risk of tuberculosis

Management

Low-risk patients with mild to moderate disease can be managed as outpatients with erythromycin, azithromycin, clarithromycin, or doxycycline (or erythromycin/sulfasoxazole in children). These agents cover *Streptococcus pneumoniae* as well as *Haemophilus influenzae, Mycoplasma pneumoniae, Legionella pneumophila,* and *Moraxella catarrhalis.* The newer macrolides (e.g., azithromycin 500 mg PO on the first day followed by 250 mg PO for 4 more days; clarithromycin every day, 500 mg PO bid for 10 days) usually are better tolerated but more expensive. Newer fluoroquinolones, such as levofloxacin (500 mg per day), are also being used more frequently. Patients with acute bronchitis don't require antibiotics.

SORE THROATS

The goals in managing a patient with a sore throat are to identify and treat streptococcal infection to prevent severe immunologic sequelae (e.g., rheumatic fever, glomerulonephritis) and to rule out life-threatening complications of pharyngeal infection.

Despite popular belief to the contrary, it is impossible to differentiate streptococcal infections from other causes of pharyngitis based on clinical grounds alone. Also, remember that most sore throats are caused by viral infections. Several epidemiologic and clinical factors increase the likelihood of streptococcal infection:

- Age > 5 years and < 15 years
- Household contacts who have streptococcal infection
- High fever, anterior cervical adenopathy, and tonsillar exudate
- Lack of signs and symptoms of systemic involvement (e.g., diffuse adenopathy, cough, runny nose, and muscular aches and pains)

Even with all the latter symptoms present, confirmation of streptococcal infections usually rests on a positive throat culture or a positive rapid streptococcal antigen assay. (These, too, can be inaccurate, but they are the best tools we have, short of serologic confirmation).

Management

A full 10-day course of antistreptococcal therapy, even without culture verification, is indicated in patients who have a history of rheumatic fever or rheumatic heart disease, recent exposure to a documented case of streptococcal infection, or a classic rash of scarlet fever.

In some hospitals, it is possible to obtain a rapid streptococcal antigen assay. A positive finding warrants antibiotic therapy without the need for a throat culture; however, a negative assay does not reliably rule out streptococcal infection and should be followed with a throat culture. If you have a high index of suspicion for streptococcal infection in patients whom you expect will have poor follow-up and compliance, a full 10-day course of therapy is warranted, even without a throat culture. In patients with a likelihood of good follow-up, you can postpone therapy until the results of the throat culture are known (usually in 2 days).

Penicillin V potassium 250 to 500 mg PO qid for 10 days

is the most specific therapy. In penicillin-allergic patients, erythromycin 250 to 500 mg or clindamycin 300 mg PO qid for 10 days is a good alternative. As the role of *Chlamydia*—recently reported in the etiology of pharyngitis—becomes clearer, erythromycin may become the therapy of choice for all patients. **PEARL: Compliance with drug therapy is enhanced by use of once-daily antibiotics.** Examples are single-dose benzathine penicillin IM and once-a-day azithromycin for 5 days and cefadroxil for 10 days orally.

Complications

Infection of the pharynx can extend into any of the potential surrounding spaces (peritonsillar, retropharyngeal, and prevertebral). If deep extension of the infection is present, urgent ENT consultation, as well as hospital admission, is required. Incision and drainage of abscesses and administration of IV antibiotics usually are indicated. Always ask the patient about difficulty breathing or swallowing (not pain on swallowing). Note whether the patient has cyanosis or any other evidence of upper airway obstruction, such as stridor.

Lateral x-rays of the soft tissues of the neck or direct fiberoptic laryngoscopy to rule out supraglottic or subglottic involvement should be performed in the stable patient with either of the following:

- A significant sore throat yet a relatively unimpressive pharyngeal examination.
- Voice changes (a voice sounding as if there is a "hot potato" in the throat) or other evidence of upper airway obstruction.

Maintaining a high index of suspicion in all cases of sore throat will help early identification and treatment of potentially life-threatening complications and adult epiglottitis. **PEARL: Severe sore throat with minimal or no pharyngeal findings suggests epiglottitis.**

SEXUALLY TRANSMITTED DISEASES

Despite the increasing fear of contracting AIDS through sexual contact, promiscuity and sexually transmitted diseases (STDs) continue to be on the rise. On encountering a patient with an STD, take advantage of the opportunity to explain to the patient how sexual transmission of diseases can be avoided. Successful management also requires concurrent treatment of sexual partners to avoid reinfection.

Male patients can present with purulent urethral discharge associated with dysuria. Female patients present with vaginal discharge, dysuria, and abdominal pain. Infections, however, can be asymptomatic in both sexes.

Historically, the most common STD has been gonorrhea. Recently, chlamydia has become increasingly prevalent. Often, concurrent infection with both organisms is present. Diagnosis is made by obtaining cultures and smears of abnormal genital discharge. A Gram's stain demonstrating gram-negative intracellular diplococci is diagnostic of *Neisseria gonorrheae* (Fig. 14–2). Treatment with ceftriaxone 125 to 250 mg IM followed by doxycycline 100 mg PO bid for 7 days will cover both gonococci and chlamydia urethritis or cervicitis. One oral dose of azithromycin 1 g can be given alternatively for chlamydial coverage and guarantees compliance. Several oral single-dose fluoroquinolone and cephalosporin options exist in addition to IM ceftriaxone. A single dose of azithromycin (2 g) is effective for treating uncomplicated gonorrhea as well as chlamydia infections. A VDRL should be obtained in all such patients, since the previously described treatment is inadequate for syphilis. Chlamydia infections also can cause painless skin lesions (e.g., ulcers, papules, nodules, vesicles) or inguinal adenopathy.

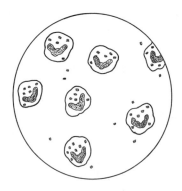

Figure 14–2. Gram-negative intracellular diplococci.

For a more detailed discussion of diagnosis and treatment of STDs, see Chapter 12. The differential diagnosis of vaginal infections is presented in Table 14–1.

Pelvic Inflammatory Disease

It is important to identify and initiate treatment for pelvic inflammatory disease (PID) as early as possible. This decreases the possibility of extension of the infection as well as late complications such as ectopic pregnancy and infertility. PID often is polymicrobial in origin, including gonococci, chlamydia, and anaerobic bacteria.

Criteria for the clinical diagnosis of PID include the presence of all of the following:

1. Abdominal tenderness with or without rebound tenderness
2. Cervical motion tenderness
3. Adnexal tenderness plus one of the following conditions.
   a. Positive Gram's stain from endocervical discharge
   b. Fever > 38°C
   c. WBCs > 10,000/mL

Indications for hospital admission include severe toxicity or sepsis and failure to respond to outpatient therapy.

Outpatient management of PID should include:

1. Ceftriaxone 250 mg IM, plus
2. Doxycycline 100 mg PO bid, *or* tetracycline 500 mg PO qid, *or* ofloxacin 400 mg PO bid for 14 days

If the patient is sent home, reevaluation within 48 hours is necessary.

DIARRHEA

Diarrhea is defined as the rapid passage of poorly formed stools. Although in the United States this is a relatively benign disease, worldwide, diarrhea still is one of the leading causes of death. The causes of diarrhea are varied; in the ED, however, most cases involve patients with infectious, viral diarrhea.

The major complications of diarrhea are dehydration and hypovolemia. Therefore, emphasis should be placed on assessing the patient's hemodynamic status. Orthostatic

Table 14–1. DIFFERENTIAL DIAGNOSIS OF VAGINAL INFECTIONS

	Normal	Bacterial Vaginosis	Trichomonas Vaginitis	Candida Vulvovaginitis
Vaginal pH	3.8–4.2	>4.5	>4.5	<4.5 (usually)
Discharge	White	Thin, homogenous, gray, adherent, increased	Yellow, frothy, adherent, increased	White, curdy, "cottage cheese"
KOH "whiff test"	Absent	Present (fishy)	May be present	Absent
Symptoms	None	Malodorous discharge, itching possibly present	Excessive discharge, foul odor, vulvar pruritus, dysuria	Itching/burning, discharge
Microscopy	Lactobacilli, epithelial cells	Clue cells, no WBCs	Trichomonads, WBCs >10/HPF	Budding yeast, hyphae, pseudohyphae

HPF = high power field; WBCs = white blood cells.

changes in the pulse and blood pressure (BP), as well as the supine vital signs, need to be measured. Dry mucous membranes, poor skin turgor, thirst, and cool peripheral extremities are additional measures of dehydration.

History

Include the following information in the patient's history:
- Description of the character of the stool (e.g., presence of blood or mucus).
- Associated symptoms such as vomiting, fever, chills, and abdominal pain.
- Epidemiologic factors: contact with patients with diarrhea, development of similar symptoms in people who shared the same meal.
- Recent travel history.
- Medication history (e.g., laxatives, antibiotics).

Always perform a rectal examination. Obtain a stool specimen and stain with methylene blue for evidence of fecal leukocytes. The presence of RBCs or WBCs suggests an invasive bacterial infection or inflammatory bowel diseases. These tests should be followed by stool cultures for bacteria and a search for ova and parasites. Guaiac-positive or bloody stools also suggest invasive diarrhea. X-rays are often not helpful but may rule out toxic megacolon or obstruction.

Management

Rehydration constitutes the cornerstone of ED management. Remember that oral rehydration often is all that is required. In fact, this is the most common form of treatment worldwide. If the patient is frankly hypotensive or is vomiting and unable to drink, establish IV access and give fluids as dictated by the clinical situation. For adults, D_5W lactated Ringer's solution or D_5W 0.45% NS with KCl 20 mEq/L and $NaHCO_3$ 50 mEq/L are additional options (considering the loss of bicarbonate and potassium in the stool). Note that KCl should be added to the fluids only after the patient voids.

Antibiotics should be given rarely in the ED and should be based on specific stool culture results (in certain infections, such as salmonella, antibiotics actually can prolong the carrier state). In adults with travel-related diarrhea, treat with a single-dose or 3-day course of a fluoroquinolone. Azithromycin is a viable alternative for treating traveler's diarrhea. Loperamide can be added in non–toxic-appearing adults. Kaopectate or Pepto-Bismol can also be given for severe cases. Arrange for a proper follow-up appointment, and have the patient return to the ED if he or she is unable to drink fluids.

MENINGITIS

Despite the wide availability of highly efficacious antibiotics, the mortality and morbidity associated with bacterial meningitis remain high. Most cases of meningitis are caused by bacteria or viruses; fungi and parasites are less common causal agents. Epidemiologic factors such as age, season, and history of exposure to a patient with meningitis help predict the causal agents. *S. pneumoniae* and *N. meningitidis* are the most common causes of bacterial meningitis in the healthy adult. *E. coli*, group B streptococci, and *Listeria monocytogenes* are seen most often in the newborn. Gram-negative rods and *L. monocytogenes* also are seen more frequently in alcoholic and immunosuppressed patients. Staphylococci should be considered in patients with a recent history of craniotomy. Early diagnosis and aggressive treatment are the keys to successful management. Therefore, all patients in whom the diagnosis of meningitis is entertained must have an immediate lumbar puncture (LP) for cerebrospinal fluid (CSF) analysis.

History and Physical Examination

Classically, patients with meningitis present with fever, headache, vomiting, photophobia, seizures, and an alteration in the mental status. On examination, many patients will be found to have neck stiffness. Clinical signs and symptoms are not always reliable in distinguishing viral from bacterial meningitis, particularly at the extremes of age and in the immunocompromised patient. This distinction requires CSF analysis. Although rare, papilledema should always be sought. Its presence suggests an increase in intracranial pressure and warrants the performance of a head CT scan before LP; otherwise, herniation could result. CT of the head also should be obtained before LP in the patients with focal neurologic findings, severe alterations in the sensorium, seizures, evidence of recent head trauma, HIV infection, and an atypical or subacute presentation.

Lumbar Puncture

An LP should be performed at the level of the L3–5 interspaces. The L3–4 interspace is found directly above an imaginary line connecting the superior surfaces of the iliac crests. In patients who can sit, this often is the easiest position for an LP, although pressures obtained can be unreliable. The lateral decubitus or "fetal" position is more practical in the debilitated patient. If you are unsuccessful with the patient in one position, it often is helpful to try changing positions. Use of a small-gauge spinal needle (#20 to #22) will help minimize the incidence of headaches. At least three 1-mL tubes should be obtained. The first tube should be sent for a Gram's stain, culture and sensitivity, and bacterial antigens. The second tube should be sent for protein and glucose. (A serum glucose should be obtained for comparison). The third tube should be sent for cell count and differential.

The differential diagnosis of meningitis based on the CSF findings is presented in Table 14–2. A traumatic bloody tap can be distinguished from bloody CSF by the absence of xanthochromia in the supernatant after centrifugation. After a traumatic tap, the true WBC count can be estimated by subtracting 1 WBC for every 500 to 1000 RBCs. Similarly, the CSF protein can be corrected by subtracting 1 mg/dL for every 1000 RBCs. Contrary to wide belief, prior treatment with oral or parenteral antibiotics has a minimal effect on the results of CSF analysis; however, cultures may be negative. Counterimmunoelectrophoresis for bacterial antigens (*H. influenzae, N. meningitidis,* and *S. pneumoniae*) can be useful and highly specific, but false-negatives are not uncommon. Bacterial antigens are particularly useful in cases of partially treated meningitis.

Management

As always, the ABCs need to be addressed initially. Active airway management, especially in the presence of seizures or altered mental status, often is required. Patients with hemodynamic compromise should be treated aggressively with IV fluids; avoid overhydration in stable patients. Patients with suspected bacterial meningitis should receive antibiotics as soon as possible. Antibiotics should never be withheld when LP is delayed (e.g., while awaiting the results of a head CT scan), but samples for

Table 14–2. CEREBROSPINAL FLUID FINDINGS

	Normal	Bacterial	Partially Treated Bacterial	Viral	Tuberculosis
Cells/mL	<5	200–5000	200–5000	<1000	<1000
Predominant cell type	Mononuclear	PMNs	PMNs	Mononuclear	Mononuclear
CSF/serum glucose ratio	0.6	Low	Low or normal	Normal	Low
Protein (mg/dL)	15–45	Very high	High	High	High
Gram's stain	Negative	Positive	Usually positive	Negative	Negative
Bacterial culture	Negative	Positive	May be positive	Negative	Negative

PMNs = polymorphonuclear leukocytes.

blood cultures should be obtained before they are administered. Sterilization of spinal fluid is rare in the first 6 hours. In the absence of a specific causal agent, a third-generation cephalosporin, such as cefotaxime or ceftriaxone 2 g IV (50 mg/kg in children), is a good initial choice. In the neonate, ampicillin 50 mg/kg IV should be added for coverage of *L. monocytogenes*. A combination of chloramphenicol and vancomycin should be used in patients with a history of severe β-lactam allergy. The use of corticosteroids, such as dexamethasone 0.15 mg/kg IV, can help prevent hearing loss if given early enough, particularly in children older than 2 months who have not received the Hib vaccine. Close contacts of patients with either meningococcal or *H. influenzae* meningitis should receive rifampin 600 mg PO (10 mg/kg in children) every 12 hours for 2 days.

All patients with suspected bacterial meningitis should be admitted and receive IV antibiotics pending culture results. Otherwise healthy patients with viral meningitis can be discharged if good follow-up is ensured.

SEPTIC SHOCK

Septic shock, if not identified and treated early, is associated with a high mortality rate. Septic shock should be suspected in any patient with a fever and hypotension, although sepsis can be present without fever in the very young or old and in the immunocompromised patient. Hypothermia may also be present.

The most common sources of septicemia are the genitourinary and gastrointestinal tracts. Therefore, gram-negative rods are the predominant organisms; gram-positive cocci, anaerobes, and fungi are other causes.

Management

Attention to the patient's ABCs is paramount. Septic shock usually is secondary to peripheral vasodilatation and can require large amounts of IV fluids. IV access should be established with at least two large-bore IV catheters, and patients should be placed on a cardiac monitor and pulse oximetry. Automated BP cuffs or an arterial line are very useful for monitoring the patient's BP. A Foley catheter should be placed in the bladder, and a urine output of at least 30 to 50 mL per hour (1 mL/kg per hour in children) should be maintained. All patients should have samples for blood and urine cultures obtained before parenteral antibiotics are administered. Any other potential sources of infection (such as sputum) also should be cultured.

Patients who do not respond to fluids need vasopressor support. We often start with a continuous IV infusion of dopamine at a rate of 2 to 20 µg/kg per minute, titrating to a systolic BP > 90 mm Hg. At rates < 5 µg/kg per minute, dopaminergic effects (renal and mesenteric vasodilatation) predominate; at levels > 10 µg/kg per minute, α-sympathomimetic effects (vasoconstriction) predominate. Patients who are unresponsive to dopamine may require IV drips with either norepinephrine 0.5 to 30 µg/minute or epinephrine 2 to 20 µg/minute.

Institute parenteral antibiotics as early as possible after pan-culturing the patient. The initial choice of antibiotics is variable and often institution-dependent. In the immunocompetent patient, cefotaxime 2 g IV is a good initial choice. A combination of ampicillin 2 g IV and gentamicin 1.5 mg/kg IV also may be given. IV drug abusers need coverage for staphylococcal species, which can be achieved with nafcillin 1 to 2 g IV. In the neutropenic or immunocompromised patient, give a combination of gentamicin 1.5 mg/kg IV and an antipseudomonal drug such as piperacillin 3 g IV or ceftazidime 2 g IV. Consider anaerobic coverage with either metronidazole 1 g IV or clindamycin 900 mg IV when an intra-abdominal source is likely. These patients are extremely ill and need to be sent to the ICU. There, the patient should have a Swan-Ganz catheter placed for proper management of fluid needs and vasopressor agents.

HIV INFECTION

AIDS has developed into a worldwide epidemic, and no matter where you work you will encounter patients with this lethal disease. Try to find out the patient's last CD4 cell count or viral load. Knowing these will help predict the clinical course. Severe immunosuppression is rare before the CD4 count falls to < 500/mL. Thrush is seen with CD4 counts between 200 and 500. As the counts fall to < 200/mL, *Pneumocystis carinii* pneumonia becomes common. Cytomegalovirus retinitis, CNS toxoplasmosis, and cryptococcal meningitis usually are seen when the CD4 count falls to < 100/ mL. Patients with AIDS usually present with one of the following complaints: fever, cough and/or dyspnea, altered mental status, and dehydration or generalized wasting.

Fever

When AIDS was first described, most patients with an HIV infection and a fever were admitted for extensive in-patient workup. With improvement in the management of opportunistic infections, many patients now are managed in the outpatient setting.

The workup of a patient with HIV infection and a fever usually includes the following:

- A thorough physical examination with particular emphasis on the degree of hydration, the lungs, and the neurologic examination
- Chest x-ray
- Pulse oximetry and/or ABGs
- CBC with manual differential
- Urinalysis and culture
- Blood cultures
- LP (in the presence of meningeal irritation or altered mental status)

The following are indications for admission of the patient with HIV infection and a fever:

- Severe dehydration not responsive to oral rehydration
- Hypoxemia
- A new infiltrate on the chest x-ray
- Evidence of meningitis or a space-occupying lesion on the head CT scan
- Neutropenia—an absolute neutrophil count (ANC) < 500 to 1000; calculate ANC as follows:

ANC = (% granulocytes + % bands) × WBC count

- Severe wasting and lack of a social support system

Shortness of Breath and a Cough

Respiratory complaints are common in patients with HIV infection. Causes include infections, neoplasms, and other idiopathic processes. Tuberculosis should always be considered present until proven otherwise. All necessary precautions should be taken, and the patient should be placed in respiratory isolation immediately. Patients with a cough or dyspnea should have a chest x-ray, ABG, sputum collection for Gram's stain, culture, acid-fast bacterial stains, and culture for tuberculosis. Calculate the patient's A-a gradient (see Chapter 2). An increased A-a gradient can be one of the earliest signs of *P. carinii* pneumonia even without significant hypoxemia. If you suspect pneumonia and cannot exclude *P. carinii* pneumonia, trimethoprim-sulfasoxazole (Bactrim) is a good antibiotic choice. Hypoxic patients with *P. carinii* pneumonia should also receive corticosteroids.

Indications for admission include hypoxemia and the presence of a new infiltrate on the chest x-ray. If you suspect tuberculosis, the patient should be admitted to an isolation bed until tuberculosis is ruled out or the patient is no longer infectious (usually after 2 weeks of antituberculous treatment).

Altered Mental Status

The workup of a patient with HIV infection should be similar to that of other patients who have an acute alteration in mental status. In addition, although not immediately indicated, a head CT scan with IV contrast should be performed on patients with HIV infection. A ring-enhancing lesion suggests toxoplasmosis or lymphoma. After excluding a space-occupying lesion and mass effect, an LP should be performed to exclude meningitis.

15

CHAPTER

Orthopedic Injuries and Swollen Joints

PREHOSPITAL CONSIDERATIONS

▶ Fractures can cause significant pain and discomfort; however, other more serious underlying injuries should always be sought.

▶ Adhere to the ABCs in all patients.

▶ Patients with long-bone injuries can lose substantial amounts of blood. If time allows, try to establish IV access en route to the hospital.

▶ Most injuries should be immobilized in the position that they are found. Gentle manipulation of extremities that are cold and without palpable pulses can be attempted.

▶ Consider administering analgesics to all stable patients in accordance with local EMS protocols.

It is beyond the scope of this chapter to review in detail all the specific orthopedic injuries and their treatment. Instead, we emphasize the general assessment and management of common orthopedic injuries. We review indications for obtaining x-rays and orthopedic consultation, and we briefly cover the use of splints. Finally, we discuss the assessment and differential diagnosis of swollen joints, with particular emphasis on recognizing the septic joint.

GENERAL PRINCIPLES

Orthopedic injuries commonly are associated with other more immediately life-threatening injuries, such as head, chest, or abdominal injuries. Therefore, the general guidelines reviewed in Chapter 3 should be applied to all orthopedic injuries as well. Also, isolated orthopedic injuries can themselves be a threat to life or limb. A femoral fracture, for example, can cause 1 to 2 liters of blood loss and hypovolemic shock.

Always begin with a rapid primary survey with assessment of the patient's ABCs. Do not let yourself be distracted by a dramatic or intensely painful orthopedic injury. Rapid resuscitation and stabilization should always precede orthopedic management.

FRACTURES

Fractures are the result of bony injury and can be open (contiguous soft tissue injury and exposure to the external environment) or closed, displaced or nondisplaced. Fractures are described in terms of the direction of the fracture line (horizontal, vertical, oblique, and spiral) and the direction and degree of angulation (always in reference to the most distal fragment). When the fracture results in more than two fragments, it is called *comminuted*.

History

Include the following information in the patient's history:
- Mechanism of injury: cause, intensity and direction of forces
- Time of injury
- Degree of resulting dysfunction (can the patient move the affected limb or ambulate?)
- History of prior injuries
- Initial treatment
- Presence of audible clicks, pops, or snaps at the time of the injury (in knee trauma, this suggests injury to the meniscus or anterior cruciate ligament)

- History of chronic illnesses, such as diabetes, renal disease, or metabolic diseases (e.g., Paget's disease)
- Occupation and hand dominance (particularly for hand injuries)

Physical Examination

To avoid errors of omission, always begin the examination with a comprehensive neurovascular assessment of the limb involved in the injury. **PEARL: Assess neurovascular status before any manipulation.** Palpate all pulses and document before you perform any manipulations. When you are unable to palpate a pulse, use a portable Doppler to assess an audible pulse. Vascular assessment also should include evaluation of skin color, temperature, and capillary refill. The neurologic examination should include assessment of sensation (pinprick in the lower extremities, two-point discrimination in the upper extremities) and motor function. Table 15–1 describes nerve injuries often associated with some of the more common orthopedic injuries.

Signs of a fracture include deformity, crepitus, swelling, ecchymosis, point tenderness, and loss of function. Only gross deformity or crepitus are definitive signs of a fracture. Always assess the entire limb as well as the adjacent joints for associated injuries. The most commonly missed fracture is a second fracture. Always assess active range of motion as well as the ability to ambulate. Don't attempt passive range of motion until you exclude a fracture.

Indications for x-rays include:

- Definite crepitus or deformity.
- Obvious dislocations.
- Significant point tenderness or swelling. **PEARL: Obtain x-rays when there is any localized tenderness or loss of function.**
- Functional impairment, including inability to bear weight or use upper extremity.
- Highly suggestive mechanism of injury.
- Neurovascular impairment.

PEARL: To assess any bony injury, take at least two x-ray views (preferably three) of injured bone and joints above and below any injuries showing trabecular detail taken at right angles to each other. When x-raying long bones, the joint above and below should be included to rule out concomitant dislocations. Contralateral comparative views can be

Table 15–1. NERVE INJURIES ASSOCIATED WITH ORTHOPEDIC INJURIES

Orthopedic Injury	Nerve Injured	Sensory Loss	Motor Weakness
Shoulder dislocation	Axillary	Deltoid region	Shoulder abduction
Humeral shaft	Radial	Dorsal 1st webspace	Wrist extension
Elbow, supracondylar	Median	Tip of 2nd finger	Thumb apposition
Elbow, lateral epicondyle	Ulnar	Tip of 5th finger	Finger abduction
Hip dislocation	Sciatic	Lateral leg and foot	Knee flexion, foot and toe flexion and extension
Knee dislocation	Tibial	Plantar foot	Foot flexion
Fibular neck	Peroneal	Lateral leg, foot dorsum	Foot extension

Table 15–2. CLINICAL GUIDELINES FOR OBTAINING RADIOGRAPHS

Ankle
- Inability to bear weight both immediately and in the ED (4 steps)
- Tenderness over the posterior tip or lower 6 cm of the distal fibula or tibia
- Young and elderly patients
- Altered mentation

Foot
- Inability to bear weight both immediately and in the ED (4 steps)
- Tenderness over the navicular bone or the base of the fifth metatarsal
- Young and elderly patients
- Altered mentation

Knee
- Inability to bear weight both immediately and in the ED (4 steps)
- Inability to flex knee to 90°
- Isolated patellar tenderness
- Tenderness at head of fibula
- Young and elderly patients
- Altered mentation

Cervical spine
- Midline cervical tenderness
- Inability to rotate head bilaterally to 45°
- Focal neurologic deficits (objective or subjective)
- Altered mentation or intoxication
- Distracting injuries (e.g., long bone fractures)

extremely helpful in difficult cases, especially in children. Clinical guidelines for obtaining ankle, knee, and cervical spine radiographs are presented in Table 15–2.

SPRAINS AND STRAINS

A sprain is an injury to a ligament (connects bone to bone); a strain is an injury to a tendon (connects muscle to bone). Sprains and strains can result in significant functional impairment and should never be brushed off as "only" a sprain or a strain. Sprains and strains are categorized according to the degree of injury.

- In *first-degree injuries,* there is mild to moderate pain and swelling over the area of the tendon or ligament with no joint laxity and minimal functional impairment.
- In *second-degree injuries,* a partial tear of the tendon or ligament results in significant pain and swelling with moderate joint laxity and functional impairment.
- In *third-degree injuries,* a complete tear of the tendon or ligament can result in minimal to significant pain and swelling, depending on whether bleeding is contained within an intact joint capsule. Significant joint instability and dysfunction are noted. Often, surgical repair is required.

INJURIES IN CHILDREN

In children, the developing growth plate is the most vulnerable element in the extremities, whereas ligamentous or tendinous injury is unusual. Therefore, with any painful injury to a bone you must rule out a growth plate fracture and treat as such. The Harris-Salter classification of epiphyseal injuries is presented in Figure 15–1. **PEARL: Injuries over growth plates should be splinted regardless of x-ray findings.** (See later discussion of splints.)

MANAGEMENT: GENERAL GUIDELINES

Reduction

Reduction of displaced fractures should be left to the orthopedist; in the presence of neurovascular compromise,

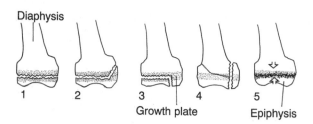

Figure 15–1. Schematic representation of the Harris-Salter classification of growth plate fractures.

however, you will be required to reduce the fracture. **PEARL: Fractures/dislocations with neurovascular compromise require immediate reduction and consultation.** A grossly displaced fracture or dislocation should be placed in an anatomic position as soon as possible. Adequate sedation and analgesia is necessary and greatly facilitates reduction. Use of short-acting reversible agents such as fentanyl 1 to 2 μg/kg IV and midazolam 1 to 4 mg IV is recommended. Close monitoring of the patient and availability of antagonistic agents (naloxone 2 mg IV and flumazenil 1 to 3 mg IV), as well as airway management adjuncts, must be ensured before sedation.

Elements of reduction include:

1. Stabilization of the proximal fragment.
2. Traction on the distal fragment along the long axis of the limb (often this alone will result in adequate reduction).
3. Reproduction of the forces that caused the initial injury.
4. Reversal of the forces that caused the injury (this is why it is so important to try to understand the mechanism and forces that resulted in the injury).

Orthopedic Consultation

Urgent orthopedic consultation should be obtained in the following circumstances:
- Displaced fracture
- Neurovascular compromise
- Most fractures in children
- Open fractures
- Unstable fractures
- Fractures that require open reduction

Patients with open fractures should receive cefazolin 1 g IV or vancomycin 1 g IV as soon as possible after a sample from the wound is cultured. Addition of an aminoglycoside (e.g., gentamycin 1.5 mg/kg IV) should be considered for open fractures with extensive soft tissue in- volvement. Tetanus prophylaxis should be considered (see Chapter 16).

Nondisplaced Fractures

You can remember how to manage nondisplaced fractures, as well as most sprains and strains, by using the mnemonic RIICE:

R rest
I ice—should be applied indirectly (have the patient apply ice cubes wrapped in plastic or cloth for 15 to 20 minutes every hour for the first 24 to 48 hours).
I immobilization—ED physicians should never apply circular casts, which can result in severe neurovascular dysfunction, especially as tissues swell. Preformed splints or those constructed from plaster of Paris or fiberglass should be used. (A more detailed description of splints follows.)
C compression—achieved by using an elastic wrap (avoid vascular compromise).
E elevation—the involved limb should be elevated above the level of the heart to facilitate venous and lymphatic drainage, which will decrease pain and swelling.

All patients with fractures and third-degree sprains and strains should be referred to an orthopedic surgeon. Telephone consultation with the surgeon before patient discharge is highly recommended.

SPECIFIC UPPER EXTREMITY INJURIES

Although a comprehensive review of all fractures and dislocations is beyond the scope of this chapter, in this section we include several "pearls" of useful information for some of the more common injuries. For further information on the diagnosis and management of specific orthopedic injuries, refer to emergency medicine or orthopedic textbooks.

Shoulder Dislocations

Most dislocations are anterior; consider posterior dislocation in patients who have had a seizure or previous shoulder injuries. On examination, you will find flattening of the shoulder over the deltoid region, prominence of the acromion, or the ability to palpate the humeral head in the subcoracoid region. Always perform neurovascular assessment. Palpate the radial pulse, and assess pinprick sensation over the deltoid region for evidence of axillary nerve injury (commonly associated with shoulder fracture dislocations).

Unless neurovascular compromise is present, obtain x-rays of the shoulder before reduction to exclude any associated fractures of the humeral head (particularly of the greater tuberosity) or of the surgical neck. The transscapular, or "Y" view, or the axillary view are particularly helpful in assessing the position of the humeral head in reference to the glenoid fossa. Sedation and analgesia (using a combination of a benzodiazepine and an opioid) are often required to facilitate reduction. We like to place the patient prone and to apply increasing traction on the outstretched arm until reduction is achieved (Stimson's technique). Superior stabilization and internal rotation of the ipsilateral scapula often helps to reduce the shoulder (Fig. 15–2). The best results are achieved by relaxing the patient's musculature with midazolam 2 to 4 mg IV.

After reduction, repeat films should be obtained to ensure adequate reduction and to rule out fractures. The shoulder should be immobilized with an arm sling, and arrangements should be made for an orthopedic follow-up examination in 1 to 2 weeks.

Radial Head Fractures

The primary bony defect is difficult to see on routine x-rays. The presence of a posterior fat pad or bulging of the anterior fat pad (the "sail sign") on a lateral view of the elbow is diagnostic of a joint effusion and, in the presence of trauma, suggests a radial head fracture (Fig. 15–3). Aspiration of blood from the radiohumeral joint with injection of a long-acting local anesthetic is very effective in alleviating the associated pain and improving mobility. The arm should be put in a sling, allowing early mobilization in 3 to 5 days. Early physical therapy is key to achieving a mobile joint.

Supracondylar Fractures of the Elbow

Supracondylar fractures in children are very serious, especially if they are displaced. They can cause vascular compromise and often are difficult to reduce. Therefore, admission is necessary. Children with nondisplaced fractures can be sent home with a reliable adult, who must be taught to monitor for signs of vascular compromise, with the appropriate immobilization.

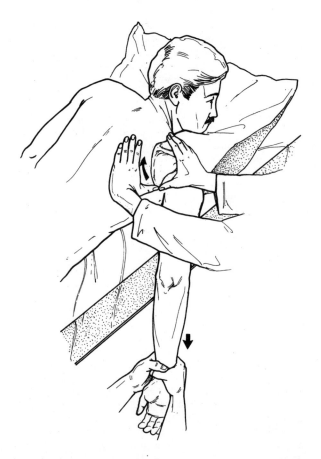

Figure 15–2. Shoulder reduction in the prone position. Traction is placed on the arm while an assistant internally rotates the tip of the scapula.

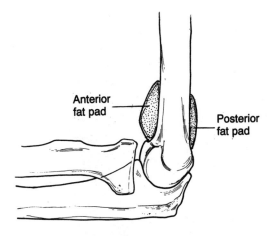

Figure 15–3. Lateral radiograph of the elbow region, demonstrating anterior and posterior fat pads.

Nursemaids' Elbow

In children under age 5 years, pulling on the outstretched arm may dislocate the radial head. The injured child presents with an immobile, partially pronated and extended elbow. Nursemaids' elbow can usually be reduced by supination and flexion of the elbow. Alternatively, pronation and flexion may be attempted. Radiographs are not routinely required.

Scaphoid Fractures of the Wrist

Scaphoid fractures usually result from a fall onto an outstretched arm and hand. They often are not visualized on routine hand and wrist films, even after a scaphoid view is obtained. Because of poor blood supply, these fractures, especially if missed, can result in malunion or nonunion. When examining the patient, apply direct pressure to the anatomic snuffbox. If tender, or if tenderness is elicited on axial compression of the thumb, suspect a scaphoid fracture and apply a thumb spica splint even if the x-ray is normal (Fig. 15–4). These injuries must be treated as if a fracture was seen on the x-ray. Orthopedic reevaluation and repeat x-ray in 10 to 14 days are necessary.

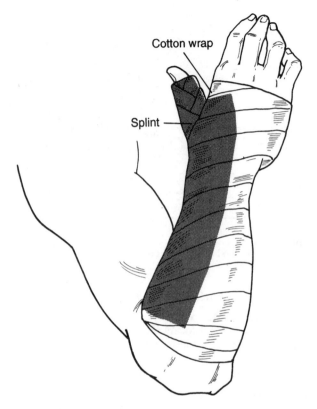

Cotton wrap

Splint

Figure 15–4. The thumb spica splint extending from the thumb-nail to the mid-forearm.

Scaphoid Lunate Dislocations

To identify scaphoid lunate dislocations, look for widening of the space between the scaphoid and the lunate >3 to 5 mm (Terry Thomas' sign).

Perilunate/Lunate Dislocations of the Wrist

In these injuries, the third metacarpal, capitate, and lunate do not line up vertically on the lateral view of the wrist. Figure 15–5 illustrates various wrist dislocations.

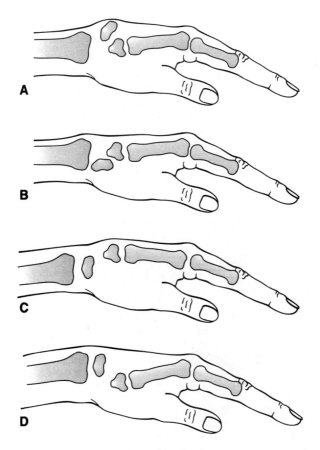

Figure 15-5. Dislocations of the wrist may take various forms, including (*A*) dorsal or (*B*) volar dislocation of the lunate, and (*C*) dorsal or (*D*) volar perilunate dislocation.

Boxer's Fractures

Fractures of the neck of the fifth metacarpal bone usually are secondary to the patient's punching a hard object. When the patient has punched someone in the face, suspect an associated human bite wound and look for a laceration. These often are deep, penetrating injuries due to the impact of the victim's teeth against the metacarpophalangeal joint. Admission for IV antibiotics and aggressive irrigation of the wound often are required. Gentle closing of the patient's fingers on the palm of your hand will demonstrate alignment of the metacarpal heads. Any angulation must be reduced. Boxer's fractures should be immobilized in an ulnar gutter splint. If there is > 30° of volar angulation or significant rotational deformity, the patient should be referred to an orthopedist. Reduction of a third or fourth metacarpal fracture is very difficult and requires orthopedic intervention.

Bennett's Fracture

Bennett's fracture is a fracture of the base of the thumb metacarpal involving the joint. Adequate reduction usually requires surgery.

SPECIFIC LOWER EXTREMITY FRACTURES

Hip Fractures

Suspect a hip fracture when a patient, especially an elderly woman, presents with an unexplained fall. On examination, the injured lower limb may appear shortened and externally rotated. Early orthopedic consultation is required for all hip fractures. Always obtain appropriate films to rule out concomitant pelvic fractures in elderly victims of a fall. X-rays may not reveal a fracture. All patients must be observed ambulating; any shuffling gait or abnormality suggests an occult fracture and requires that additional films be taken (e.g., a "frog's leg" Judet's view). An MRI of the hip can be obtained in highly suspicious cases with normal plain films.

Hip Dislocations

Hip dislocations are most frequently posterior and often are associated with knee injuries because of the mechanism of injury (i.e., usually a force applied against the flexed knee with the hip in flexion). The leg usually is shortened and in internal rotation. Early reduction is necessary to avoid avascular necrosis of the femoral head. Injury to the sciatic nerve must always be excluded.

Knee Injuries

Knee injuries can be accompanied by significant swelling, making it difficult to diagnose specific ligamentous or meniscal injuries at the time of injury. A complete knee evaluation may be required 5 to 7 days later when the swelling has decreased. A tense, painful, traumatic knee effusion should be evacuated. The presence of fatty globules in the joint indicates an intra-articular fracture (e.g., a tibial plateau fracture). Knee immobilization and crutches for ambulation should be given to patients with significant pain or inability to bear weight on the injured knee. A follow-up examination with an orthopedist within 1 week is recommended. Radiographs should be obtained as indicated in Table 15–2.

Patients with knee dislocations have a high incidence of accompanying popliteal arterial injury; thus, arteriography should be performed in these patients.

Ankle Sprains

In addition to examining the ankle for swelling, tenderness, deformity, and instability, palpate the fifth metatarsal as well as the *proximal* fibula for evidence of associated injuries. A complete neurovascular examination should always be included. If radiographs are indicated (Table 15–2), the base of the fifth metatarsal should always be included in the film. This can rule out an avulsion fracture (traction by the peroneus brevis muscle) or a true Jones' fracture (a transverse fracture through the distal fifth metatarsal diaphysis where both cortices appear thickened). Radiographs of the foot should also be considered (Table 15–2).

SPLINTS

Splints, not circumferential casts, are the preferred method of immobilization in the ED. Splints can be useful in the following conditions: fractures, sprains, strains, joint infections, arthritis, tenosynovitis, lacerations that cross joints, deep space infections, and puncture wounds of the hands and feet. **PEARL: Use splints in all patients with significant discomfort.**

Plaster of Paris is a cloth impregnated with dextrose or starch and a semihydrated calcium sulfate. When water is added to the plaster of Paris, crystallization occurs, resulting in an exothermic reaction (which is more rapid and severe when hotter water is used; so use lukewarm water). Use between 8 and 12 layers of plaster. Cover the limb with stockinet to protect the skin; then wrap the limb with a single layer of soft cotton (Webril) to create padding, which further protects the skin and bony prominences and allows for swelling.

Measurement of splint length should be made over the corresponding contralateral limb. Immerse the plaster of Paris in lukewarm water until all air bubbling ceases. Express excess water by wringing the plaster between your index and middle fingers. Apply the plaster to the affected limb, smoothing it out with the palms of your hands (the plaster should conform loosely to the limb). As the plaster hardens, apply a circumferential elastic or gauze wrap starting at the most distal level. Each wrap should overlap 50% of the prior wrap. Leave the distal end of the limb exposed to allow assessment of color and temperature. Fold back the end of the stockinet over the splint to create a smooth, padded edge. The plaster hardens within 15 to 30 minutes, but it continues to set for 24 hours, during which time weight bearing should be avoided.

SWOLLEN JOINTS

There are many causes of swollen joints, but in the absence of trauma, your main objective is to identify patients with a septic joint. Staphylococcal, gonococcal, and pneumococcal organisms are the most common causes of septic arthritis and can rapidly destroy a joint if not quickly diagnosed and treated. If you can't rule out a septic joint, arthrocentesis must be performed.

History

In gathering information from the patient, ask the following questions:
- If multiple joints are involved, was there an additive or migratory pattern to the involvement?
- Are there associated symptoms such as a fever, chills, or rash?
- Is there any history of STDs?
- Is there any history of trauma?

Physical Examination

When performing the examination, ascertain the following:

- Is the joint hot, red, and swollen—or just swollen?
- Are there signs of generalized toxicity, such as fever, tachycardia, or hypotension?
- Are there signs associated with systemic lupus erythematosus, such as a malar rash, alopecia, or pharyngeal ulcers?

Gonococcal arthritis is suggested by the presence of discrete purplish papules over the extensor surfaces of the fingers, tenosynovitis, and/or a cervical or urethral discharge.

Laboratory Tests

The most important test is a joint aspiration, which must be performed in all patients with an atraumatic swollen joint in whom the possibility of septic arthritis is considered. Indications for arthrocentesis include:

- A solitary red or hot joint
- Monoarticular or oligoarticular involvement in the presence of fever or chills

Joint fluid should be obtained under strict sterile conditions and sent for CBC and differential, glucose, Gram's stain, crystals, and culture and sensitivity. Note that joint aspiration is contraindicated in the presence of overlying skin infection. Table 15–3 classifies the various types of arthritis based on synovial fluid findings.

If septic arthritis is present, obtain blood cultures as well as throat, cervical, urethral, and rectal cultures. In the absence of septic arthritis, the following labs may be indicated: erythrocyte sedimentation rate (ESR), antinuclear antibody (ANA), rheumatoid factor, antistreptolysin titer, Lyme titer, and C-reactive protein.

Children with a suspected septic hip should be evaluated with ultrasound.

Septic Arthritis

Patients with septic arthritis can present with abrupt onset of a red, hot, swollen joint. The most commonly involved joints are the knees, hips, and wrists. Often, these patients have associated fever and chills. Gonococcal arthritis, the

Table 15–3. CLASSIFICATION OF ARTHRITIS BASED ON SYNOVIAL FLUID ANALYSIS

	Normal	Noninflammatory	Inflammatory	Septic	Traumatic
Clarity	Transparent	Transparent	Transparent-opaque	Opaque	Opaque
Color	Clear	Yellow	Yellow-white	Yellow	Pink
Viscosity	High	Low	Low	Low	High
WBCs/mL	< 200	200–3000	3000–75,000	> 75,000	< 200
% PMNs	< 25	< 25	> 50	> 75	< 25
Glucose	= Serum	= Serum	< Serum	< Serum	= Serum

PMNs = polymorphonuclear leukocytes; WBCs = white blood cells.

most common cause of infection, often is associated with a periarticular tenosynovitis, particularly around the anatomic snuffbox. As previously noted, typical skin lesions may be found.

If septic arthritis is a possibility, empirical IV antibiotics, such as cefotaxime 1 to 2 g IV, must be started as soon as joint and blood cultures have been obtained. All patients with septic arthritis should be admitted to the orthopedic service.

16

CHAPTER

Principles of Wound Management

PREHOSPITAL CONSIDERATIONS

▶ Most lacerations are not life-threatening; however, other associated injuries must be excluded by performing a primary survey following the standard ABCs.
▶ Hemostasis should be achieved using direct manual pressure or pressure dressings.
▶ Elevation and splinting of the injured area will help stop bleeding and reduce patient discomfort.

The ultimate goals of wound management are to restore function and achieve an optimal cosmetic result. Infection, which develops in approximately 3% of wounds, adversely affects these goals. Therefore, meticulous care should be given to minimize this complication.

HISTORY

The following information should be obtained from all patients.

- **When did the injury occur?** As more time elapses, the degree of bacterial contamination increases. It is commonly taught that if more than 6 to 12 hours have elapsed (the "golden period" of the wound), it is unwise to close the wound. In areas of good vasculature (e.g., face, scalp), however, the tissues' ability to resist infection is greater, and wounds can be closed up to 24 hours after the injury. Even in areas of good blood supply, if the wound appears highly contaminated, either excise the wound margins (thus creating a new wound if excess tissue is available) or defer wound closure for several days. (This is called *delayed primary closure.*)

- **What caused the injury?** Injury with a dirty, potentially contaminated object increases the likelihood of infection. Mammalian bites (e.g., dogs, cats, humans) increase the risk also.
- **Is there any possibility of retained foreign bodies? PEARL: Always inquire about potential foreign bodies.** Foreign bodies are present in approximately 3% of wounds and increase the risk of infection. Regular soft tissue x-rays, ultrasound, CT scanning, or even MRI can help identify a foreign body. Probe all wounds manually for the presence of foreign bodies. (If sharp foreign bodies are likely, use an instrument to probe the wound.) Glass, the most common foreign body, usually is seen on regular x-rays regardless of its lead content. A skin marker and at least two views will help you to determine where the foreign body is.
- **Was the wound cleaned after the injury?** What was used to clean the wound?
- **When did the patient last receive a tetanus shot?** Table 16–1 presents the current recommendations concerning the need for both passive [tetanus immune globulin (TIG)] and active [tetanus-diphtheria toxoid (Td)] tetanus prophylaxis. **PEARL: Give TIG in inadequately immunized patients with tetanus-prone wounds.**
- **Does the patient have any underlying immunocompromising conditions** (e.g., cancer, diabetes, steroid use, chemotherapy, AIDS)?
- **Is the patient allergic to antibiotics?** (This will affect your choice of antibiotics, if indicated.)
- **Is the patient allergic to local anesthetics?**
- **Is the patient allergic to latex products?** This is more common in health care workers and patients with spina bifida. If so, avoid all latex products.

Table 16–1. RECOMMENDATIONS
FOR TETANUS PROPHYLAXIS

	Clean Minor Wounds		All Other Wounds	
	Td	TIG	Td	TIG
History of tetanus immunization				
Doses, uncertain to < 3	Yes	No	Yes	Yes
Doses ≥ 3	No*	No	No†	No

*Yes, if more than 10 years since last dose.
†Yes, if more than 5 years since last dose.
Td = tetanus-diphtheria toxoid; TIG = tetanus immune globulin.

PHYSICAL EXAMINATION

Adequate examination and management of a wound usually require local anesthesia. Always perform and document a complete neurovascular examination before giving an anesthetic. Evaluate pulses and capillary refill distal to the injury. In the hand, two-point discrimination (using a paper clip bent in two) is the best sensory modality to be examined. Elsewhere, evaluate pinprick sensation. **PEARL: Exclude nerve and tendon injuries in all extremity wounds.** Check range of motion to evaluate for tendon or ligament injury and muscle strength. An adequate examination requires good lighting and a relatively bloodless field. Temporary placement of tourniquets can be helpful in extremity lacerations.

WOUND PREPARATION

The cornerstone of wound management includes mechanical debridement of devitalized tissue and copious irrigation with a balanced physiologic solution, such as normal saline (NS).

Local Anesthesia

Local anesthetics (which stabilize cell membranes) are either esters or amides. An easy way to remember to which group a particular anesthetic belongs is to note that all amides have the letter "i" in their generic name before the suffix "caine" (e.g., lidocaine, mepivacaine). The importance of knowing the chemical class of a particular agent stems from the fact that most allergic reactions to local anesthetics are due to the esters or the methylparabate preservative used in lidocaine preparations. If a true allergy to lidocaine is present, you can use the parenteral form of diphenhydramine diluted 1:4 with NS or benzoyl alcohol (the preservative in multidose saline vials) as a local anesthetic. The most commonly used local anesthetics are lidocaine and bupivacaine. Their onset, duration, and toxic ranges are presented in Table 16–2.

The addition of epinephrine to the local anesthetic causes vasoconstriction, resulting in improved hemostasis, decreased systemic absorption, and prolonged action. Epinephrine should be avoided in the digits, tip of nose, and tip of penis (think "nose, toes, fingers, hose").

PEARL: Topical anesthetics should be used to reduce the pain of infiltration. To decrease the pain caused by infiltrating a local anesthetic, take the following steps:

- Apply a topical anesthetic (lidocaine, epinephrine, and tetracaine) before injecting the anesthetic.
- Use a small needle, preferably #27 gauge.
- Inject as slowly as possible.
- Dilute lidocaine 10:1 with sodium bicarbonate 8.5% IV solution (this diluted product has a shelf life of at least 1 week)
- Warm the local anesthetic to body temperature.
- Pinch the skin adjacent to the wound just before injecting the local anesthetic.
- Inject the local anesthetic into the subcutaneous plane instead of the intradermal plane (this has a longer onset but is much less painful).

Table 16–2. CHARACTERISTICS OF LIDOCAINE AND BUPIVACAINE

Anesthetic Agent	Onset (min)	Duration	Acceptable Safe Total Dose
Lidocaine	2–5 min	30–120 min	4–5 mg/kg
Bupivacaine	5–10 min	4–8 h	2–3 mg/kg

- In clean wounds, insert the needle through the wound edges. (If the wound is contaminated, it is better to infiltrate the skin around the wound.) Enter at one end and slowly infiltrate the anesthetic around the wound in continuous circular advancements, so the patient will feel only one needle stick (Fig. 16–1).

Irrigation

Irrigation has been shown to be effective in removing both bacteria and infection-potentiating factors, such as soil, from the wound. The efficiency of irrigation increases with higher pressures and volumes of fluid. **PEARL: Use a plastic shield when irrigating to minimize splatter.** We suggest using

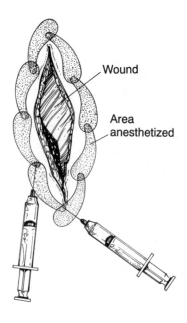

Figure 16–1. Anesthetizing the wound. The wound is anesthetized in a circular motion. With each successive injection, the needle enters a previously anesthetized area.

a 35- or 65-mL syringe with a plastic shield. A minimum of 100 mL of crystalloid per 1 cm of wound should be used.

After adequate irrigation, the wound and its surrounding edges should be scrubbed with a dilute 1% povidone iodine (Betadine) solution (do not use the scrub solution intended for prepping operative fields in the operating room). Do not irrigate the wound with alcohol, hydrogen peroxide, or concentrated povidone iodine solution.

Debridement

Devitalized, crushed, avascular tissue forms an excellent medium for bacterial growth. **PEARL: Remove as much devitalized tissue as possible.** Adequate debridement sometimes requires the use of local flaps or grafts for closure of the remaining defect. In these cases, it probably is best to consult the plastic surgeon. Vital tissues such as nerves and tendons, however, must be preserved.

WOUND CLOSURE

There are several options for wound closure, each with different advantages and disadvantages (Table 16–3). The most commonly used method for closing wounds is suturing. Choice of the appropriate suture material should be based on the suture's characteristics and intended uses (Table 16–4). For facial lacerations, a 5/0 or 6/0 suture is appropriate; for most finger lacerations, use a 5/0 suture. For all other lacerations, a number 4/0 suture may be used.

PEARL: Appropriately used tissue adhesives save time and reduce discomfort. A new tissue adhesive, octylcyanoacrylate (Dermabond, Ethicon), recently received FDA approval. It is an excellent choice for closure of noncontaminated wounds under minimal tension, particularly on the face and torso. Butylcyanoacrylate is an alternative for short superficial wounds, particularly on the face, but it is not yet FDA-approved. Compared with butylcyanoacrylate, octylcyanoacrylate is three times stronger, more flexible, and transparent (Fig. 16–2).

Tissue adhesives slough off after 7 to 14 days. Patients should not scrub or soak their wounds but may wet them. Don't place ointments and adhesive tapes on the adhesive. Remember, just because you choose a tissue adhesive doesn't mean that a full wound evaluation and preparation are no longer required.

Table 16–3. COMPARISON OF WOUND CLOSURE METHODS

Method	Advantages	Disadvantages	Recommended Uses
Sutures	Considerable experience Allows most meticulous closure Greatest breaking strength Lowest dehiscence rate	Requires anesthesia Requires removal Greatest tissue reactivity Highest cost Time-consuming Risk of needlestick	Complex lacerations Lacerations subject to considerable tension Deep closure
Staples	Rapid application Ease of use Low tissue reactivity Reduced risk of needle stick	Less meticulous closure Patient discomfort Requires removal May interfere with imaging	Scalp and torso lacerations Multiple trauma Temporary closure
Tissue adhesives	Rapid application Ease of use	Lower tensile strength than sutures	Facial and torso lacerations Extremity lacerations under minimal tension

	Advantages	Disadvantages	Comments
	May not require anesthesia Patient comfort No need for removal No risk of needle stick Resists bacterial infection	Higher initial cost Not good for hair-bearing areas	May be used in conjunction with deep sutures in lacerations subject to tension Closure of superficial lacerations subject to no tension
Surgical tapes	Least tissue reactivity Lowest infection rates Patient comfort Low cost Rapid application Ease of use No risk of needle stick	Lowest tensile strength Highest dehiscence rate Use of toxic adjuncts to improve adhesiveness required Cannot be used in hair-bearing areas Must remain dry	Usually in conjunction with deep sutures Good for reinforcing lacerations after suture or staple removal

Table 16-4. SUTURE CHARACTERISTICS

Suture	Knot Security	Tensile Strength	Duration of Wound Security (days)	Tissue Reactivity	Recommended Uses
Nonabsorbable					
Nylon (Ethilon)	Good	Good	NA	Minimal	Percutaneous closure Tendon repairs
Polypropylene (Prolene)	Fair	Excellent	NA	Minimal	Percutaneous closure Tendon repairs
Silk	Excellent	Fair	NA	Most	Percutaneous closure
Absorbable					
Surgical gut	Poor	Fair	5–7	Moderate	Mucous membranes
Chromic cut	Fair	Fair	10–14	Moderate	Mucous membranes
Polyglactin (Vicryl)	Good	Good	30	Minimal	Deep sutures
Irradiated polyglactin (Vicryl Rapide)	Good	Good	10–14	Minimal	Percutaneous or mucosal closure in children
Poliglecaprone (Monocryl)	Good	Good	30	Minimal	Deep sutures
Polyglycolic acid (Dexon)	Excellent	Good	30	Minimal	Deep closure
Polydioxanone (PDS)	Fair	Excellent	45–60	Slight	Deep closure under significant tension
Polyglyconate (Maxon)	Fair	Excellent	45–60	Slight	Deep closure under significant tension

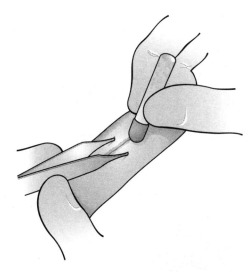

Figure 16–2. Application technique for a tissue adhesive.

Helpful Tips for Wound Closure

- Tie your knots just enough to approximate wound edges. **PEARL: Don't tie sutures too tightly; this will strangulate the tissues and cause necrosis and sloughing of the edges.** (Remember that tissue swelling will increase during the next 24 to 48 hours.)
- Take equal "bites" from both sides of the wound. More tissue should be taken at the depth of the wound than at the surface (Fig. 16–3).
- Try to evert the wound edges. If you have difficulty doing this, use a vertical mattress suture (Fig. 16–4). Sometimes, it is useful to alternate simple with mattress sutures to achieve eversion yet save time.
- If one side of the wound is longer than the other side, use wider spaces between adjacent sutures on the longer side. This may prevent the formation of a "dog ear" at the end. The management of a dog ear is illustrated in Figure 16–5.
- The length of the suture ends should be roughly equal to the distance between adjacent sutures. Don't cut the sutures too close to the end. This makes suture removal more difficult.

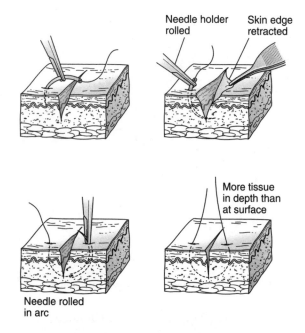

Figure 16–3. Placement of a simple suture. By holding the needle upside down and excessively pronating the wrist, the needle tip moves farther away from the laceration with deeper penetration. Thus, more tissue is at the depth of the wound, causing eversion of the wound edges.

- Facilitate closure of scalp wounds by tying knots in the hair to keep wound edges together.
- **PEARL: Use deep sutures for all gaping wounds subject to tension to avoid dehiscence and wide scars (Fig. 16–6). Undermining of wounds may help closure.**

Wound Dressings

Most wounds should be covered with an antibiotic ointment, such as bacitracin, and a dry gauze or adhesive bandage (Band-Aid). Wounds closed with a tissue adhesive can be covered with a dry dressing; however, avoid application of any ointments. In areas of hair, bacitracin alone is adequate. By the way, the purpose of shaving hair

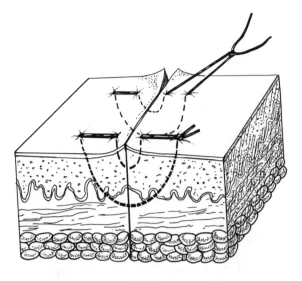

Figure 16–4. Vertical mattress sutures for approximation and eversion of skin edges.

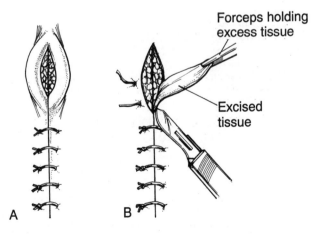

Figure 16–5. Correction of a "dog ear." (*A*) Dog ear. (*B*) Excision of dog ear with closure of defect.

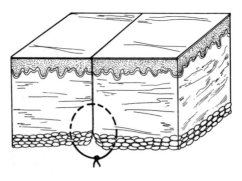

Figure 16–6. Deep suture. Note that the knot is buried in the depth of the wound.

around the wound is to facilitate wound closure, not to reduce wound infection. In fact, it can increase the risk of wound infections. The use of hair clippers is preferred. Never shave the hairs of the eyebrow.

Suture or Staple Removal

The timing of suture removal usually can be determined by wound location:
- Face: 3 to 5 days
- Extremities and digits: 10 to 14 days
- Trunk: 10 days
- Elsewhere: 7 days

PEARL: After suture removal, reinforce the wound with surgical tapes to reduce the risk of dehiscence or wide scars.

PATIENT INSTRUCTIONS FOR WOUND CARE

The following instructions should be given to all patients:
- Keep the wound clean and dry. After 24 to 48 hours, the wound may be washed gently and then covered with a clean dressing.
- If the wound is on an extremity, elevate the extremity for 48 hours to reduce swelling.
- Return to the ED if there is increasing swelling, red-

ness, or pain around the wound; yellow or green discharge from the wound; fever; or shaking chills.

INDICATIONS FOR CALLING A PLASTIC SURGEON

Always let the patient (or his or her parents) know that a scar is unavoidable yet can always be corrected at a later date (usually after at least 6 to 12 months), if necessary. A plastic surgeon should be consulted in the following circumstances:

- When the wound involves the lacrimal apparatus or the canthal ligaments of the eye.
- When tissue loss is extensive, requiring grafting or complex local flaps other than simple undermining of the wound edges.
- When lacerations involve the corner of the mouth or the philtrum ("Cupid's bow").
- When the patient or family insists that you call a plastic surgeon.

ANTIBIOTICS

Prophylactic antibiotics are not routinely indicated. A list of generally accepted indications for prophylactic antibiotics is presented in Table 16–5.

The risk of contracting rabies is greatest in cases of raccoon, bat, and skunk bites. It is unlikely in rodent bites. Rabies has been reported with aerosol exposure, especially from bats. In cat or dog bites, ask about the immunization status of the pet. If the rabies immunization status is unknown, suggest that the animal be observed by the owner for 10 days. Contact the local health department for suspicious bites. In cases of exposure to an animal suspected to have rabies, give human rabies immune globulin 20 U/kg (half around the wound, half IM) plus human diploid cell vaccine 1 mL IM immediately, then 1 mL IM on days 3, 7, 14, and 28. Rabies vaccine absorbed can also be given instead of the human diploid cell vaccine—1 mL IM immediately, then 1 mL IM on days 3, 7, 14, and 28.

Table 16–5. PROPHYLACTIC ANTIBIOTICS

Type of Wound	Common Organisms	Indications for Prophylaxis	Antibiotic Regimens
Human bite	Streptococci Staphylococci *Bacteroides* *Eikenella corrodens*	All bites with break in skin	Augmentin 875/125 mg PO BID Clindamycin 300 mg PO BID plus Cipro 500 mg BID or Bactrim in children Consider admission and IV antibiotics with injuries over metacarpophalangeal joints
Dog bite	*Pasteurella multocida* Streptococci Staphylococci	All extremity bites Extensive injuries Deep puncture wounds	As above
Cat bite	*P. multocida* Staphylococci	All bites	As above
Bat, raccoon, skunk	Unknown	All bites	Augmentin 875/125 mg PO BID Doxycycline 100 mg PO BID

17
CHAPTER

Environmental Disorders

BURILS

PREHOSPITAL CONSIDERATIONS

> ▸ All patients require 100% O_2 via nonrebreather mask.
> ▸ Cool burns with cold water, then cover with a sterile or clean sheet.
> ▸ Avoid excessive cooling with ice, especially with burns over a large area.
> ▸ Do not cover burned skin with any creams or ointments.
> ▸ Chemical burns require copious irrigation.

Burns are the result of thermal injury and are caused by scalding fluids, steam, fire, electricity, or chemicals. In the past, fluid loss was a major cause of mortality; today, inhalational injury and sepsis are the major contributing factors. Therefore, in addition to aggressive fluid management, early recognition of inhalational injury and appropriate management are paramount. Remember, too, that the patient may also have other significant injuries and should be managed as for any other multiply injured patient.

The prognosis of burn victims depends on the patient's age, the extent of the burn [percentage of body surface area (% BSA)], the burn depth, the presence of associated inhalational injury, and the patient's past medical history. Therefore, every one of the latter factors must be assessed.

History

Include the following information in the patient's history.
- What caused the injury?
- What kind of material was combusted?
- Did the injury occur in a closed space?
- Is there any evidence of inhalation injury?
- Was the patient conscious at the scene?
- What treatment was already given at the scene and en route (e.g., O_2, fluids)?
- Does the patient have any underlying medical illnesses or immunocompromised conditions?

Initial Assessment and Management of the Burn Victim

Airway

Immediately determine whether there are any signs of present or impending airway compromise. Facial edema, singed nasal vibrisae, perioral burns, and carbonaceous sputum should all increase your degree of suspicion of inhalational injury. Laryngeal edema can develop rapidly, making endotracheal intubation very difficult or impossible. **PEARL: Assume all patients with flame injuries in a closed space have an inhalation injury and may need immediate intubation.** Therefore, if there is any suggestion of airway compromise, intubate the patient with the largest endotracheal tube possible. If there already is significant laryngeal edema making intubation impossible, perform a cricothyroidotomy

Breathing

Inhalational injury secondary to toxic fumes or steam as well as carbon monoxide or cyanide poisoning should always be suspected. All patients should receive 100%

supplemental O_2 while ABGs and carboxyhemoglobin levels are being obtained. For a more detailed review of carbon monoxide and cyanide poisonings, see Chapter 11. Patients who fail to maintain adequate oxygenation (PaO_2 60 mm Hg on 100% O_2) or ventilation ($PaCO_2 > 50$ mm Hg) require intubation and mechanical ventilation.

Circulation

Burns cause significant external fluid loss as well as large internal fluid shifts. Rapidly assess the patient's hemodynamic stability. **PEARL: Establish IV access with at least two large-bore IV catheters, preferably through intact skin (IVs can be placed through injured skin if no other sites are available).** Femoral lines or saphenous venous cutdowns present a high risk for infection or thrombosis and should be avoided. Monitor urine output closely using an indwelling urethral catheter.

Fluid Resuscitation

The patient's fluid requirements during the first 24 hours can be estimated with the Parkland formula.

2 to 4 mL/kg of lactated Ringer's lactate per % BSA (up to 50%) burned should be given during the first 24 hours (only second- and third-degree burns should be considered in calculating percentage of BSA). Half of the requirements are given within the first 8 hours from the time of the injury (*not* from the time of presentation). Make adjustments based on clinical parameters, such as vital signs, urine output, and central venous pressure.

Assessment of the Burn

Depth

Burns are classified according to depth:
- **First-degree burns** involve only the epidermis, causing erythema and pain.
- **Second-degree burns** involve the epidermis and part of the dermis, causing blistering and severe pain.
- **Third-degree burns** involve the epidermis and all elements of the dermis as well as subdermal tissues.

They are characterized by coagulation of blood vessels and white or brown, shiny, leathery skin. These burns do not blanch and usually are not painful because the nerves are destroyed.

Percentage of Body Surface Area

This can be estimated roughly by using the patient's palm, which equals 1% of the total BSA, as a reference. In adults, use the "rule of nines":

Head = 9%
Anterior trunk = 18%
Posterior trunk = 18%
Upper limb = 9%
Anterior lower limb = 9%
Posterior lower limb = 9%
Genitalia = 1%

In children, the head is larger and the lower limbs smaller in proportion to adults (Fig. 17–1).

Local Treatment of Burns

In third-degree burns, eschars (necrotic burned tissues) are stiff and, if circumferential, can compromise circulation (in the limbs) or breathing (in the trunk). **PEARL: If there is any evidence of vascular or respiratory compromise, perform an escharotomy.** Use a #10 scalpel along the sides of the arms, legs, digits, or chest as required (Fig. 17–2). Anesthesia is not necessary, and the incision should be deep enough to allow the scar to expand and the subcutaneous fat to bulge, thus improving circulation or ventilation.

Cleanse second-degree burns with a balanced crystalloid solution. Ruptured blisters should be gently debrided; however, unruptured blisters should be left intact. Then, cover the burns with a sterile dressing. If the patient is to be discharged, use an antimicrobial cream such as bacitracin or silver sulfadiazine.

Disposition

Indications for admission to the hospital include:
- Second-degree burns covering > 10% BSA.
- Third-degree burns covering > 5% BSA.

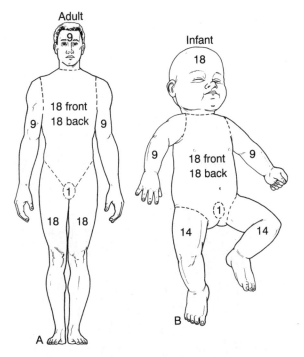

Figure 17–1. The "rule of nines" for calculating the body surface area in an adult *(A)* and a child *(B)*.

- Burns involving the hands, feet, eyes, ears, or perineum.
- High-voltage electrical burns.
- Significant underlying illnesses.
- Extremes of age (infants < 1 year of age, elderly > 65 years).
- Suspected child abuse. **PEARL: Consider child abuse with scald burns, especially in children < 3 years old.**

All wounds should be reevaluated within 48 hours. Systemic antibiotic prophylaxis is not indicated. Give tetanus prophylaxis in accordance with the guidelines presented in Chapter 16.

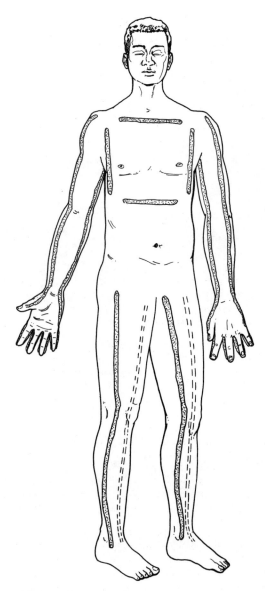

Figure 17–2. Performing escharotomies.

COLD INJURIES
Hypothermia

PREHOSPITAL CONSIDERATIONS

▶ Handle patients gently and place cardiac monitor immediately.
▶ Do not perform CPR in patients in whom you don't feel a pulse if they have a viable cardiac rhythm.
▶ Start two large-bore IVs and hydrate with warm normal saline.

Hypothermia is defined as a body temperature < 35°C and can result from multiple factors leading to increased heat loss, decreased heat production, or impaired thermogenesis due to central mechanisms. The most common cause of severe hypothermia is ambient exposure. The most common of the numerous predisposing conditions are alcohol ingestion, hypoglycemia, sepsis, hypothyroidism, and hypoadrenalism.

Hypothermia is classified by the degree of core temperature reduction:

1. **Mild hypothermia:** 32.5°C to 35°C
2. **Moderate hypothermia:** 27.5°C to 32.5°C
3. **Severe hypothermia:** <27.5°C

The first response to hypothermia is shivering, which effectively generates heat by increasing the metabolic rate two to five times. As glycogen stores are depleted and the body temperature reaches 30°C, this response is lost. Other responses to cold exposure are vasoconstriction and diuresis, which contribute to the shock state.

Alcohol ingestion often is a confounding factor because it increases heat loss by vasodilatation and enhances diuresis while altering a person's judgment as to the need to wear protective garments.

Hypothermia may affect many systems:

• **Cardiovascular:** An initial tachycardia is followed by a progressive and severe bradycardia secondary to a decrease in the spontaneous firing rate of the cardiac pacemaker cells (this is why bradycardia secondary to hypothermia is usually refractory to standard treatment such as atropine). The most characteristic ECG abnormality in patients with hypothermia is the J wave (Osborn wave) or hypothermic hump (Fig. 17–3). Most commonly, this appears at temperatures < 25°C, yet can be seen at temperatures < 32°C.

- **CNS:** Cerebral metabolism decreases approximately 6% to 7% for each degree of temperature change between 25°C and 35°C, and the EEG becomes flat at approximately 20°C. Deep tendon reflexes often are lost at temperatures < 30°C. Confusion followed by lethargy is common.
- **Renal:** Diuresis is followed by a drop in renal blood flow, causing a profound hypovolemia.
- **Respiratory:** Respirations become slow and shallow.

Management

The most important factor in management of hypothermia is early recognition and rapid rewarming of the patient. **PEARL: Start to rewarm the patient immediately except for a frozen extremity—leave it frozen** (see "Frostbite"). Although detection of hypothermia is simple, the diagnosis often is missed in the ED. Staff may fail to measure temperatures at all, especially in resuscitations (note: if a resuscitation effort is not succeeding, check the patient's core temperature). In addition, be sure to check the temperature of all patients with an altered mental status or irrational behavior (especially the elderly patient). Another reason for missing hypothermia is the thermometer itself. Many thermometers, even electronic ones, fail to detect temperatures < 34.5°C. Always use special hypothermia thermometers.

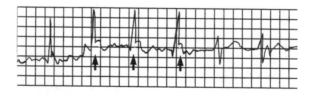

Figure 17–3. Hypothermic J waves.

Resuscitation should begin, as always, with assessment of the ABCs and the usual care of any patient with an altered mental status (see Chapter 7 for more details). Stabilization of the ABCs (with intubation and ventilation as required) and IV insertion should be followed by administration of glucose (as indicated by a Dextrostix), thiamine, and naloxone. If the patient is in ventricular fibrillation, attempt to defibrillate three times only, although antiarrhythmic drugs and electrical defibrillation rarely are effective before the patient is warmed. Intubate as gently as possible, since intubation may theoretically induce ventricular fibrillation. Place a Foley catheter and gastric tube in all patients.

Obtain blood samples for toxicology screen, coagulation profile, creatinine phosphokinase (CPK) levels, thyroid function tests, CBC, cortisol, and ABGs (measured ABG values rather than corrected values should be used for patient care).

Rewarming Methods

- **Passive external warming** consists of placing the patient in a warm environment, providing warm clothing, and allowing the body to regain heat. This treatment is limited to patients with *mild hypothermia*.
- **Active external rewarming** involves the external application of heat such as hot water bottles, warm blankets, or even immersion in a tub of warm water. It is indicated for patients with *moderate hypothermia* when more advanced facilities are unavailable.
- **Active core rewarming** is the application of heat into the core or central parts of the body. Warmed inhaled oxygen is the simplest method. Esophageal or rectal lavage with warmed fluids also can be performed (avoid irrigating the area containing the temperature probe). More invasive methods include peritoneal lavage, pleural lavage, femoral-arteriovenous bypass, and cardiopulmonary bypass (either full or partial) using warmed fluids. Active core rewarming is appropriate for patients with *severe hypothermia* or those with *hemodynamic impairment*.

PEARL: A patient should never be pronounced dead until *warm and dead.* All resuscitative efforts should be continued until the patient's core temperature reaches 32°C.

Frostbite

PREHOSPITAL CONSIDERATIONS

▸ Remove any cold or wet garments or shoes and cover the patient with warm blankets.
▸ Leave frostbitten limbs frozen until a definitive rewarming method is available.

Frostbite is a form of local tissue injury due to freezing cold, whereas *trench foot* occurs with prolonged exposure to wet (yet nonfreezing) cold temperatures. The most commonly involved areas are those farthest from the body core with the poorest blood supply, such as the feet, hands, nose, earlobes, and cheeks. Predisposing factors include alcohol or other vasodilating drugs, malnutrition, anemia, poor local circulation, and cigarette smoking.

Frostbite is divided into superficial and deep injuries. In superficial frostbite, large clear blisters (resembling a second-degree burn) appear, followed by hardening and darkening of the skin. Beneath the surface, however, the skin remains soft and pliable. In deep frostbite, the tissue is deep purple or red with hemorrhagic blisters and is cool to the touch. Sensation and distal function are often absent, and the tissues feel hard like wood or stone.

Early prediction of the severity of injury is very difficult, and partial or full recovery may be the result of an initially necrotic-appearing limb. Therefore, any decisions concerning surgical treatment should be delayed until clear demarcation is apparent, approximately 6 months later.

Management

PEARL: Treat hypothermia. Wet or cold garments should be removed immediately. Avoid excessive manipulation of frostbitten extremities. Rapid rewarming of the frozen part is the most important measure. **PEARL: Thawing of injured areas may be extremely painful—give adequate analgesia.** Rewarming can be achieved by immersing the injured tissue in 42°C circulating water until a distal flush of the extremity is noted. Dry heat can be very dangerous and should be avoided. Recently, aloe vera (a selective inhibitor of thromboxane A_2), together with an oral NSAID such as ibuprofen, has been suggested as an effective local treatment for frostbite. Hemorrhagic blisters should be left alone, but clear blisters probably should be debrided. Although systemic antibiotic prophylaxis is not indicated, local antibiotics such as bacitracin or silver sulfadiazine can be used. Involved extremities should be elevated, and cotton should be placed between the toes and fingers. Tetanus prophylaxis should be considered and administered as described in Chapter 16.

Indications for hospital admission include:

- Concomitant hypothermia
- Any immunocompromised diseases
- Significant facial involvement
- Bilateral extremity frostbite
- Deep frostbite injuries
- Frostbite involving most of one limb

HEAT INJURIES

PREHOSPITAL CONSIDERATIONS

▶ Establish IV access and hydrate with fluids.
▶ Institute rapid cooling methods as available (spraying with cool water or application of ice packs, removal or loosening of clothing, ensure proper air circulation or use of air conditioning).

Heat Stroke

Heat stroke is a condition characterized by failure of central thermoregulation; patients present with a high temperature (usually defined as $> 41°C$) and an altered mental status. **PEARL: Consider heat stroke in all patients with an altered mental status, particularly after exertion.** In the past, it was believed that heat stroke was always associated with anhidrosis, but young patients with exertional heat stroke may present with diaphoresis.

Remember that the patient's temperature may have fallen spontaneously or because of cooling before arriving at the ED. Therefore, do not exclude a heat stroke based on the initial ED temperature reading. Also, it is very important to rule out other life-threatening causes of hyperthermia, including sepsis, meningitis, stroke, brain tumors, head injuries, and withdrawal from substances of abuse. Be wary of heat strokes especially during hot, humid weather and in patients who collapse after extreme physical exertion. **PEARL: A core temperature should be obtained early in all patients with an altered mental status.**

History

In obtaining the patient's history, ask the following questions:

- Did the symptoms follow strenuous physical activity?
- Were the symptoms concurrent with headaches, stiff neck, or vomiting?
- Does the patient have a history of any disorders that interfere with sweating and, therefore, heat loss (e.g., icthyosis, psoriasis)?
- Is the patient taking any medications that can predispose to heat stroke, such as diuretics, β-blockers, antiparkinsonian drugs, neuroleptic agents?

Assessment

- Begin by assessing the ABCs. Patients with heat stroke who are unconscious or lethargic may need to be intubated to protect their airway.
- Since patients with heat stroke often are dehydrated, establish IV access and start fluid resuscitation as required.
- Check a Dextrostix and give $D_{50}W$ 50 mL by IV push if the glucose level is low, in addition to thiamine and naloxone, as you would for all patients with an altered mental status.
- Accurate measurement of the core temperature with a rectal probe is necessary for early recognition and treatment.
- Examine the patient for evidence of an infectious disease, head injury, or stroke.
- Draw blood for CBC, Chem 7, prothrombin time (PT), partial thromboplastin time (PTT), ABGs, creatine phosphokinase, and urinalysis.

Myoglobinuria is common and should be treated with alkalization of the urine and forced diuresis. **PEARL: The presence of dark urine may indicate myoglobinuria and rhabdomyolysis requiring aggressive diuresis and alkalinization.** Disseminated intravascular coagulation (DIC) can occur and should be treated with coagulation factors (i.e., fresh frozen plasma) and platelet replacements as necessary.

Treatment

Cooling the patient as quickly as possible forms the cornerstone of treatment. Patients who are alert and hemodynamically stable can be placed in a tub filled with cold water or ice. If a tub is unavailable or the patient is not stable, spray him or her with water mist and place the patient under a high-speed fan. Aggressive cooling should be continued until the patient's temperature falls to < 38.5°C (note: avoid overshooting and causing hypothermia). Fluid and electrolyte imbalance should be corrected as the clinical condition warrants. **PEARL: All patients with heat stroke need to be admitted.**

Heat Exhaustion

Patients with heat exhaustion present with dehydration, nausea and vomiting, muscle cramps, and sometimes confusion. Their temperature is only moderately elevated. IV replacement of fluid and salt repletion with a balanced isotonic solution often is required. This condition often is seen in poorly acclimatized patients who exert themselves in hot, humid climates. If severely dehydrated, these patients must be admitted.

Heat Cramps

Heat cramps are caused by depletion of sodium caused by extreme physical exertion and sweating. Patients can be afebrile and complain of muscle cramps. They should be treated with replacement of water and sodium losses, and most can be discharged. Patients should be encouraged to continue to consume large amounts of salt-enriched fluids at home, such as Gatorade or other mineral drinks.

NEAR DROWNING

PREHOSPITAL CONSIDERATIONS

▶ Consider hypothermia in all drowning victims.
▶ Consider C-spine injuries in all drowning victims, and immobilize patients with stiff collar and backboard.
▶ Support ABCs with oxygen, and assist ventilation, if required.

Drowning is defined as death from suffocation after submersion in water, whereas *near drowning* refers to survival after submersion. *Delayed drowning* or *secondary drowning* occurs when a patient who was apparently doing well after surviving submersion suddenly deteriorates. There is a bimodal distribution of those at risk, patients under 3 years of age and teenagers. Alcohol and drug abuse plays a significant role in many drowning and near-drowning cases, especially among youths. In submersion accidents involving diving injuries, concomitant cervical spine injuries are common and must be excluded. **PEARL: Rule out spinal injuries in all victims of drowning.** Myocardial ischemia, seizures, and hypothermia may also be factors in submersion accidents and should always be considered. In approximately 15% of cases, laryngospasm causes death due to asphyxia, referred to as "dry drowning."

In the past, much emphasis was put on differentiating between freshwater and saltwater drowning. In most cases, however, the quantity of aspiration is not large enough to cause significant electrolyte shifts or hemolysis; *hypoxemia* is the major cause of morbidity and mortality. Hypoxemia can result from surfactant washout (leading to atelectasis), ventilation-perfusion mismatch, or damage to the alveolar capillary membrane. Noncardiogenic pulmonary edema can result from direct pulmonary injury.

History

In obtaining the patient's history, ask the following questions.

- How long was the patient under water?
- What was the temperature of the water?
- Did the patient require resuscitation?

- Was there a diving/shallow water injury?
- How soon did resuscitation begin?
- Does the patient have any underlying diseases, such as ischemic heart disease, seizures, or diabetes?
- Was there any evidence of drug or alcohol ingestion before the accident?

Management

Assessment of the patient's ABCs with C-spine precautions and immobilization should be performed as soon as the patient arrives at the ED. **PEARL: Obtain pulse oximetry and a chest x-ray in all but asymptomatic patients.** Always look for associated injuries or underlying causes. **PEARL: All patients need supplemental O_2.** Patients who are obtunded or who remain hypoxic ($PO_2 < 60$) despite O_2 therapy must be intubated and mechanically ventilated. Patients often require positive end-expiratory pressure (PEEP) to achieve adequate oxygenation. Hypotensive patients should receive aggressive fluid resuscitation, but central venous pressure monitoring may be required to avoid overhydration and pulmonary edema. Measure a rectal or esophageal temperature to rule out hypothermia, which may be either the cause or the result of the near drowning. The following labs should be obtained: C-spine, CBC, Chem 7, PT, PTT, urinalysis, ECG, ABGs, and a chest x-ray. Note that the chest x-ray may or may not be helpful early on; often, radiologic findings lag behind changes in the ABGs. A nasogastric tube should be placed to empty the stomach and to avoid any further aspiration. Placement of a urethral catheter will help monitor urinary output. Repeated boluses of sodium bicarbonate (1 mEq/kg IV push) should be given, as required, for metabolic acidosis (pH < 7.10). Antibiotics and steroids are not indicated. Arrhythmias, which often result from hypoxia and acidosis, should be treated with appropriate antiarrhythmics.

Indications for Admission

All patients who are hypoxemic and require O_2 must be admitted to the hospital. Asymptomatic patients without evidence of significant submersion can be discharged. Asymptomatic patients who have had a significant submersion or mildly symptomatic patients should be observed in the ED for several hours and can be discharged if their chest x-ray and oxygenation level remain normal.

18

The Difficult Patient

PREHOSPITAL CONSIDERATIONS

▶ Consider hypoglycemia and obtain a Dextrostix in all violent patients.
▶ Police assistance may be required for transport of violent patients.

The "difficult patient" arouses feelings of animosity and hostility in the health care provider. Such patients include those who are verbally or physically abusive, intoxicated, suicidal, homeless, malodorous, and self-abusive. Often, the health care provider has negative feelings either before he or she meets the patient, based on the nurse's report or the patient's chief complaint, or immediately upon entering the patient's room. These patients, however, need your attention most. **PEARL: Remember that the patient's abnormal behavior may be the result of a serious underlying disease, even in psychiatric patients.** Also, because of their social isolation, these patients are at risk for developing many serious illnesses. Therefore, a thorough evaluation is always required. The somnolent alcoholic patient lying in your ED may simply be drunk, but also might be suffering from a subdural hematoma, hypoglycemia, or a brain abscess. **PEARL: Exclude hypoglycemia in all violent patients.**

THE VIOLENT PATIENT

It is always best to try to identify potentially violent patients before they actually become violent. **PEARL: Predictors of violence include male gender, drug or alcohol abuse, and history of violence.** The following are conditions in which violent behavior should be anticipated:

- Alcohol or drug abuse
- Acute psychotic or manic disorder
- History of violent behavior
- Antisocial personality
- Severe psychomotor agitation (e.g., pacing, yelling)
- Restraints already in place or patient brought in by police

PEARL: Potentially violent patients require rapid attention, which often helps to diffuse their anger. All angry patients should be considered potentially violent. These patients should be isolated from other patients and visitors. Offering a comfortable chair or food may help. Never argue with a potentially violent patient. Also, never touch the unrestrained violent patient before obtaining permission, and always stand at least an arm's length away.

Physical Restraint

An actively violent patient must be restrained for his or her own protection from serious injury, as well as for the protection of the health care providers. Carefully document in the patient's chart why the restraint was necessary. Restraining the patient also facilitates patient evaluation, which might otherwise be impossible. Never turn your back on or stay alone in a closed room with a potentially violent patient. Leave the door open, and do not stand in the way if the patient attempts to bolt out of the room. Also, always leave yourself an easy avenue of exit. Some patients, if placed in a quiet environment, can be "talked down." In other instances, a show of force is enough to subdue a potentially violent patient.

Enter the room with confidence, and explain to the patient in a strong, steady tone that you are there to help. If the patient refuses to stay calm, say you will need to use a restraint. Usually, at least five people are required to physically restrain a violent patient. Each member of the team should be assigned one limb, and all members should approach the patient simultaneously. The patient should then be put into a strong four-point restraint and a posey (a thick cloth device intended to restrain the trunk). Placing patients on their side helps to prevent aspiration, although the supine position with elevated head is more comfortable and facilitates the examination. Explain to the patient that you are using a restraint to avoid further injury to anyone. All violent and suicidal patients should be searched for weapons (which may be concealed in their undergarments).

Chemical Restraint

Physical restraints usually are sufficient, but often the violent patient requires a chemical restraint as well, such as a major (neuroleptics) or minor (benzodiazepines) tranquilizer. This protects the patient from injuries (e.g., rhabdomyolysis) due to struggling against the restraint and can facilitate evaluation.

Neuroleptics are particularly effective, having relatively few side effects such as cardiorespiratory depression. Haloperidol 5 mg IV or IM every 10 to 20 minutes is used most commonly. Note that IV use of haloperidol is not yet approved by the FDA. Droperidol, which has a more rapid onset and fewer adverse reactions than haloperidol, also can be given in doses of 2.5 mg IV or IM every 10 minutes. All neuroleptics can cause an acute dystonic reaction, which should be managed with diphenhydramine 50 mg IV or benztropine 2 mg IV.

Benzodiazepines can cause respiratory depression, yet are safer to use when seizures are a possibility (e.g., in those with alcohol withdrawal, antidepressants, cocaine abuse). Lorazepam 1 mg IV or IM every 5 to 10 minutes or midazolam 0.5 to 1.0 mg IV can be given as needed. If you choose benzodiazepines, be prepared to intubate the patient if necessary. Use a cardiac monitor and pulse oximetry to monitor the patient. Frequent reassessment of the patient is required. **PEARL: Rapid chemical restraint may be obtained by combining a butyrophenone with a benzodiazepine.** A combination of lorazepam 2 mg and haloperidol 5 mg or droperidol 2.5 mg is more effective than either drug alone.

Differential Diagnosis

The differential diagnosis of violent behavior can be remembered by the mnemonic FIND ME, as shown in Table 18–1.

Table 18–1. DIFFERENTIAL DIAGNOSIS OF VIOLENT BEHAVIOR: FINDME

Functional disorders
  Schizophrenia
  Paranoia
  Mania
  Antisocial or borderline personality disorders
  Post-traumatic stress disorder
Infections
  Meningitis
  Encephalitis
  Sepsis
Neurologic disorders
  Head injuries
  Seizures (especially temporal lobe)
  Postictal state
  Neoplasms
  Vasculitis
  Dementia
Drug-related disorders. **PEARL: Consider a drug reaction, especially in the elderly.**
  Alcohol intoxication or withdrawal
  PCP (phencyclidine)
  Cocaine
  Amphetamines
  LSD (lysergic acid diethylamide)
  Anticholinergics
  Opioid withdrawal
  Sedative hypnotic withdrawal
  γ-Hydroxybutyrate
Metabolic disorders
  Electrolyte abnormalities
  Acute renal or hepatic failure
  Hypothermia or hyperthermia
  Hypoxia
  Vitamin deficiencies
  Hypertensive encephalopathy
Endocrine disorders
  Hypoglycemia
  Thyroid storm
  Cushing's disease

Workup

Extensive workup is indicated in the violent patient with a suspected organic cause. Table 18–2 presents several findings to help distinguish organic from functional causes of violence. **PEARL: Abnormal vital signs, disorientation, altered mental status, and lack of psychiatric history suggest an organic cause of violence.**

The following tests should be considered in the workup: CBC, electrolytes, renal function tests, liver function tests, osmolarity, CT scan of the head, lumbar puncture (LP; especially if the patient has fever or signs of meningeal irritation), ethanol level, and urine toxicology screen or blood toxicology (or both).

After underlying medical conditions are ruled out, violent patients should be seen by a psychiatrist.

THE INTOXICATED PATIENT

An alcoholic patient presenting with an altered mental status may be suffering from any of the following conditions:
- Acute intoxication with ethanol or mixed substances such as methanol, ethylene glycol, and/or cocaine.

Table 18–2. COMPARISON OF FINDINGS IN FUNCTIONAL AND ORGANIC DISORDERS

	Functional	Organic
Age of onset	15–45 yr	Any age
Acuity	Days to weeks	Acute
Prior psychiatric history	Often present	Often absent
Vital signs	Usually normal	Often abnormal
Physical examination	Usually normal	Often abnormal
Level of alertness	Usually normal	May be abnormal
Orientation	Usually normal	Often abnormal
Speech	Normal or pressured	Often abnormal
Delusions	Often present	Absent
Hallucinations	Auditory	May be visual or tactile
Memory	Usually normal	Often abnormal short-term

- Subdural hematoma or any other intracranial structural lesion.
- Hypoglycemia, ketoacidosis, or electrolyte imbalance.
- CNS infection.
- Thiamine deficiency with acute Wernicke's encephalopathy.
- Delirium tremens.
- Any other medical problem unrelated to intoxication.

All known alcoholic patients or patients with alcohol on their breath who present with an altered mental status should undergo a thorough physical examination to rule out any significant underlying diseases. Ascertain the following:

- Is there evidence of trauma?
- Is there nuchal rigidity?
- Is the patient febrile?
- Are there focal neurologic findings or signs of increased intracranial pressure?
- Were there any focal or new-onset seizures?

All intoxicated patients should have a rapid glucose determination by a Dextrostix. Consider obtaining a blood alcohol level. Most patients with an altered mental status should receive thiamine 100 mg IVP, $D_{50}W$ 50 mL IV (if glucose is low or unmeasurable), and naloxone 2 mg IV as indicated. Continue to reassess these patients every 15 to 30 minutes for signs of deterioration. If the patient's blood alcohol level is not high, immediately proceed with an extensive workup for an altered mental status including blood labs, head CT, toxicology screen, and possibly an LP (see Chapter 4).

Indications for an urgent head CT in alcohol-dependent patients include:

- Focal or new-onset seizures
- Evidence of head trauma
- Signs of increased intracranial pressure or focal neurologic findings on examination
- An unimproved or deteriorating level of consciousness

If the initial alcohol level is high and the patient's level of consciousness improves, usually no further workup is necessary. As a rough estimate, non–alcohol-dependent patients metabolize alcohol at a rate of 15 to 20 mg/dL per hour. In alcohol-dependent patients, the metabolism is enhanced, and the clearance increases to 25 to 30 mg/dL per hour. **PEARL: Remember that alcohol-dependent patients may have very high blood alcohol levels while acting completely sober.**

THE HOMELESS PATIENT

Because of poor nutrition and hygiene, inaccessible medical care, and lack of social supports, otherwise benign illnesses can develop a malignant course among the homeless. Also, these patients tend to present for treatment much later in the course of their disease and, therefore, often have a more serious illness. Soft tissue infections, pneumonia, and dehydration (which might other- wise be managed outside the hospital) can require inpatient care because of poor patient compliance and lack of stable medical follow-up.

Lack of adequate shelter exposes the homeless to the extreme elements and their associated conditions, such as frostbite, trench foot, hypothermia, heat exhaustion, and heat stroke. Therefore, a rectal temperature should be measured, especially during the cold months. Other commonly encountered problems in the homeless include malnutrition, skin ulcers, lice, scabies, alcohol abuse, trauma, viral hepatitis, tuberculosis, and mental illnesses.

If the patient is being discharged, a follow-up should be arranged. We recommend using social services to help arrange for proper disposition. If no alternative care is possible, have the patient come back to the ED for a follow-up.

19
CHAPTER

Ethical, Social, and Legal Issues in the Emergency Department

PREHOSPITAL CONSIDERATIONS

- The ambulance provides a safe environment in which it is possible to separate the victim from the abuser.
- Accurate documentation is important, especially when the patient refuses transport.
- Request police assistance with disoriented or violent patients who refuse transport.
- Ask about any DNR orders, health care proxies, or living wills before instituting resuscitative efforts or leaving the patient's home.

Although an exhaustive (and exhausting) treatise on medical ethics and legal medicine is beyond the scope of this chapter, it will help you to have some familiarity with basic legal and ethical principles. For all of these issues, be sure to discuss problems with the attending physician, social worker, and/or ethics consultants if they are available in your hospital, because the laws and protocols vary from place to place. In this chapter, we cover three issues: patient consent and leaving against medical advice, DNR (do not resuscitate) orders and living wills, and domestic violence and rape.

CONSENT AND COMPETENCE

Two of the major guiding principles of medical ethics are *beneficence* (helping, or at least not harming, the patient) and *autonomy* (the right of every mentally competent adult to control his or her body). Autonomy requires that we obtain consent from patients to examine and treat them. Usually, this is not a problem; occasionally, however, a patient refuses treatment, forcing us to decide whether we can treat this person against his or her will. To examine this a little more closely, look at the types of consent we usually obtain for treatment.

Express consent means that a person specifically agrees to a particular examination or procedure. Legally, this must be *informed consent* as well, meaning that the person has had the risks and benefits of the action, and alternative actions, explained before giving consent. Any time a procedure is done on a patient, it is good medial practice to obtain this type of consent. *Implied consent* is the situation in which a person, by his or her actions, can be assumed to have given consent (e.g., rolling up his or her sleeve when told that blood needs to be drawn). The doctrine of *emergency consent* is frequently encountered in the ED; it covers the situation in which the patient is unable to give consent but requires life-saving treatment. The standard of care is to assume that the patient would consent in that situation to those procedures that a "reasonable person" would consent to.

The giving of consent assumes a capable adult patient. The legal and ethical principles of autonomy hold that any patient can refuse any examination or treatment. (Note that competency is a legal definition, ruled on by a judge. Physicians, including psychiatrists, cannot truly define someone as competent or incompetent to make decisions, although this is routinely and quite necessarily done in practice. What is actually being assessed, as termed by the legal system, is the "capacity" to make judgments.) Consent for a minor must be given by a capable adult who is the legal guardian. Note that this is not always the parent! If consent is not immediately available for a minor, the prevailing standard is for the physician to carry out care that is necessary to preserve life or limb, or to prevent the patient's condition from worsening. The problems that arise if a minor's guardian actually refuses to consent to a procedure that the physician deems necessary are beyond the scope of this chapter. No minor or child can sign out against medical advice if there is a life-threatening condition. If such a situation arises, discuss it with the attending physician and the hospital legal consultant.

As noted, competent adults are able to refuse any treatment. If such a person does wish to leave the ED, he or she must be permitted to go. It is up to the physician to determine who has capacity to make decisions. Occasionally, EM physicians request a psychiatric consultation to determine capacity. In general, these patients must be alert; oriented to self, time, and place; and must demonstrate by reciting back to you that they understand the risks of leaving. The patient must not have any psychiatric disease that would impair judgment; especially, he or she must not be suicidal. Document in the chart that you have explained these risks; be specific about what they are. Have the patient, and preferably an accompanying person such as a spouse, sign that note or an against medical advice (AMA) form, if one exists at your institution. Sometimes, a patient refuses to sign anything. In this case, be especially sure that this person is competent by your assessment, document extremely thoroughly, and have someone sign the note as a witness to the patient's refusal to sign. **PEARL: If any doubt exists regarding the capacity of an unstable patient to refuse medical care, he or she should not be allowed to leave against medical advice.**

RAPE, ASSAULT, DOMESTIC VIOLENCE, AND ABUSE

A legal issue that often arises is the intersection of the ED with the criminal justice system. The physician is bound by specific legal requirements. Specific situations that arise are rape, assault, and suspected child or elder abuse. Always notify the attending physician when one of these situations arises.

Rape

The crime of rape is violent and traumatic with long-term psychological consequences. It is imperative that the horror of the event doesn't include the victim's treatment in the ED. Have a social worker or a community ED companion immediately available to help the patient get through the medical evaluation.

The initial evaluation must be directed to the patient's physical well-being. Injuries must be treated as for those of any other patient. Approach the patient in a nonthreatening and reassuring manner. Always have an assistant present who is of the same sex as the victim. Once immediate physical problems are dealt with, get a brief history of the attack. Document the general appearance and the patient's demeanor and physical findings appropriately on the chart, with particular attention to bruises and marks. Use a body map to describe the bruises. Obtain permission and take photographs of any marks or bruises, especially if the patient hasn't involved the police yet. Ask the patient if he or she wishes to involve the police. Using a rape evidence kit facilitates the physical examination. Follow local protocols for its use. The patient should receive STD prophylaxis, hepatitis virus vaccination, HIV prophylaxis, and postcoital contraception according to CDC recommendations (Table 19–1).

Although not all experts agree, most patients probably benefit from prophylaxis because (1) follow-up of patients who have been sexually assaulted can be difficult and (2) patients may be reassured if offered treatment or prophylaxis for possible infection.

Make appropriate referral for counseling and follow-up.

Assault

In the case of a victim of assault, again, the medical care of the patient is paramount. Because of the legal issues, the H&P should be documented meticulously. As with rape cases, ascertain if the victim wants the police to be involved, and make any such arrangements. Certain states require EDs to report felony assaults (e.g., gunshot wounds, knife wounds). Patients should be referred for counseling as well.

Abuse

In the ED, always maintain a high degree of suspicion of abuse. **PEARL: Screen all women for risk of domestic violence.**

Table 19–1. STD PROPHYLAXIS AND POSTCOITAL CONTRACEPTION IN RAPE CASES

Drug	Dosage
STD prophylaxis	
Ciprofloxacin	500 mg PO once
Plus	
Azithromycin	1 g PO once
Plus	
Metronidazole	2 g PO once
HIV prophylaxis	
Combivir (zidovudine 300 mg and lamivudine 150 mg)	1 tablet PO BID for 4 weeks
Plus	
Indinavir	800 mg PO TID for 4 weeks
Postcoital contraception (within 72 hours of coitus only if pregnancy test currently negative)	
Norgestrel (Ovral)	2 tablets PO [or (Lo/Ovral) 4 tablets PO]; repeat dose in 12 hours

All ages are susceptible to being abused, although children, women, and the elderly are more likely to be victims. As always, medical care is paramount. Whenever you do suspect abuse, you should notify the appropriate agencies; this usually is a legal requirement for physicians. Often, if not always, the hospital's social work department should be involved. Although many women who are victims of abuse will not volunteer any information, they will discuss it if asked simple, direct questions in a nonjudgmental way and in a confidential setting. **PEARL: Ask every woman if anyone has hurt her or hit her or if she is afraid to go home because of violence.** You may want to offer a statement such as: "Because violence is so common in many women's lives, I've begun to ask about it routinely." Then, you can ask a direct question, such as: "At any time, has your partner hit, kicked, or otherwise hurt or frightened you?" *If the patient answers yes, the following steps are suggested:*

1. Encourage her to talk about it.
2. Listen nonjudgmentally.

3. Validate her visit to the ED. Victims of domestic violence are frequently not believed, and the fear they report is minimized. Tell her that what happened to her is a crime and that help is available for her.
4. Document the patient's complaints and symptoms as well as the results of the observation and assessment and detailed description of the injuries, including type, number, size, location, resolution, possible causes, and explanations given.
5. Assess the danger to your patient and the patient's safety before she leaves the medical setting.

Treat the patient's injuries as indicated. In prescribing medication, keep in mind that medications that hinder the patient's ability to protect herself or to flee from a violent partner may endanger her life. *If the patient answers no or will not discuss the topic, be aware of clinical findings that may indicate abuse:*

- Injury to the head, neck, torso, breasts, abdomen, or genitals.
- Bilateral or multiple injuries.
- Delay between onset of injury and seeking treatment.
- Explanation by the patient that is inconsistent with the type of injury. **PEARL: Suspect domestic violence when the history is not consistent with the injury.**
- Any injury during pregnancy, especially to the abdomen or breasts.
- History of trauma.
- Chronic pain symptoms for which no etiology is apparent.
- Psychological distress, such as depression, suicidal ideation, anxiety, and/or sleep disorders.
- A partner who seems overly protective or who will not leave the woman's side.

If any of the above clinical signs are present, it is appropriate to ask more specific questions.

A woman is most at risk of serious injury or even homicide when she attempts to leave an abusive partner, and it may take her a long time before she can finally do so. It is frustrating for the physician when a patient stays in an abusive situation. Be reassured that if you have acknowledged and validated her situation and offered appropriate referrals, you have done what you can to help her.

HEALTH CARE PROXY, LIVING WILLS, AND "DO NOT RESUSCITATE" ORDERS

Patient autonomy can continue even after a person is no longer competent to give or refuse consent. **PEARL: Try to obtain information regarding presence of DNR orders, advance directives, and living will before resuscitative efforts, especially in terminally ill patients.** Some examples of this are health care proxy forms, living wills, and DNR orders. These are extremely relevant in the ED setting. In general, what these instruments do is legally limit the types of care to be given to the patient. The document names a health care proxy, a person who is legally assigned to make health care decisions for the patient. This allows the named person the full legal right to make medical decisions as if it were the patient directly. Be aware that a DNR order means just that: "Do not resuscitate." That means, do not attempt any interventions if the patient is pulseless. It does *not* mean to withhold antibiotics, food, water, or even pressor agents in some cases. A health care proxy may make those decisions. The DNR order also may not apply to certain circumstances, such as after a suicide attempt. A living will generally is broader in nature; often it discusses the patient's desires about specific therapies but does not have the legal clout of a health care proxy. If you have any doubt about a patient's supposed wishes, such as when you have only a companion's verbal statement that a person is a DNR, you are ethically and legally obligated to treat that patient as most people would wish to be treated (i.e., resuscitate). Although this may result in the resuscitation of a person who did not wish this, such an action is far better than allowing a patient to die who would have wanted the resuscitation attempt to be made. Note that a patient can revoke a DNR order at any time merely by saying so.

THE DEATH OF A PATIENT

One of the hardest psychosocial situations you will face in the ED is informing a family of a patient's death, especially the death of a child. In general, you should have the family members placed in a separate and quiet room, preferably with a phone available. Have someone go in with you, such as a nurse, social worker, or member of the clergy.

Usually, the attending physician should be with you as well for at least part of the discussion. Be direct but supportive. Use the word "dead"; euphemisms such as "passed away" or "didn't make it" may not get the message across. Always tell the family that you did everything you could. If possible, assure them that the death was painless and that their relative didn't suffer. After you have told them, stay in the room as long as needed to answer their questions.

If the family is not present, it is best not to tell them over the telephone. Instead, tell them that their relative is critically ill and that they ought to come in. Tell them to drive safely and make sure they know how to get to the hospital.

Depending on the laws and procedures in your hospital, you may have to bring up the subjects of autopsy and organ donation to the family of the deceased. Almost any patient may be a candidate for tissue donation. This can be very difficult, but it often is helpful to explain that such procedures allow the deceased to help others. For autopsy, point out that the information obtained may answer the family's questions about the cause of death and provide useful medical information for relatives about inherited diseases (including cardiovascular disease). After you leave, someone should remain with the family to help them make funeral arrangements and inform other family members. Note that some deaths, varying from place to place, especially unexpected deaths, fall under the jurisdiction of the medical examiner or coroner. In these cases, you may be required to contact that official, and the family then must be informed that their relative may be legally required to undergo an autopsy.

Finally, remember to deal with your own feelings about the death. Don't hesitate to talk to coworkers, friends, social workers, clergy, or counselors if you are troubled. Many resources exist to help you deal with the legal, social, and ethical difficulties that crop up in the ED. Clergy often are on call for patients who need or request them. They can help a family to deal with the stress of a death or serious illness or to face decisions such as DNR status. The social work service of your hospital may have a full-time or on-call social worker; this person should be involved in all cases of possible abuse or neglect and can be an additional support for families facing the stress of illness. Consider them also for patients with primarily social problems, such as the homeless. Also consider them for patients who may have psychosocial difficulties in addition to their medical problems, such as the elderly, patients with substance abuse problems, or patients with financial trouble that may compromise their care (e.g., preventing them from filling prescriptions). Keep in mind that you are not alone, and use the help available to you.

TAKING CARE OF YOURSELF

Throughout your work in the ED, keep yourself healthy. Get as much sleep as possible, eat appropriately, exercise regularly, and maintain your friendships and family relationships. Avoid alcohol, tobacco, and other harmful substances. Take care of yourself properly so you can take care of others properly.

A

APPENDIX

*Advanced Cardiac Life Support Algorithms**

---

*Source: Circulation [2000;102(suppl I):I-158–I-165 and I-172–I-203]. © 2000 American Heart Association, Inc., with permission.

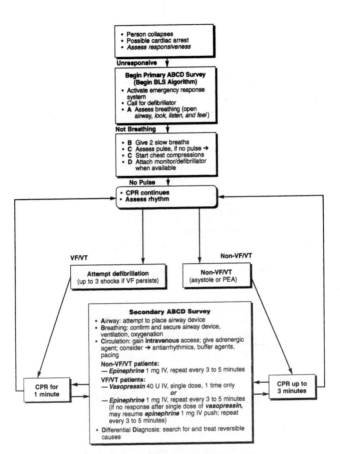

Figure 1. Comprehensive ECC Algorithm.

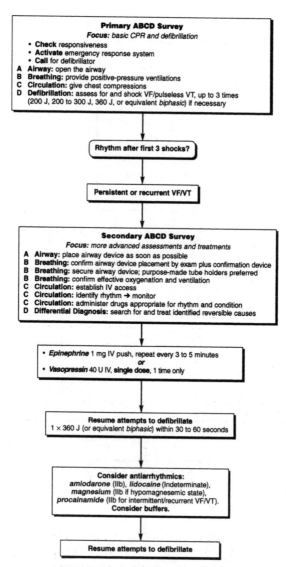

Figure 2. Ventricular Fibrillation/Pulseless Ventricular Tachycardia (VT) Algorithm.

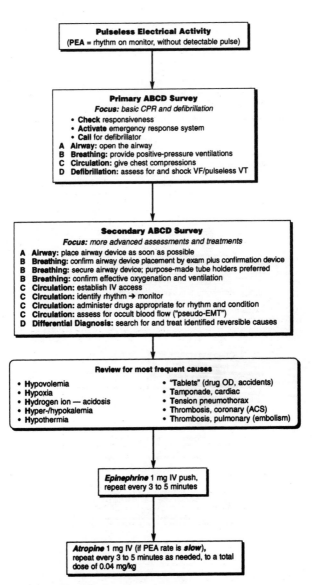

Figure 3. Pulseless Electrical Activity Algorithm.

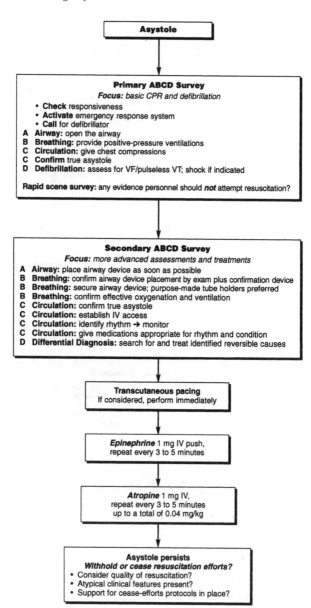

Figure 4. Asystole: The Silent Heart Algorithm.

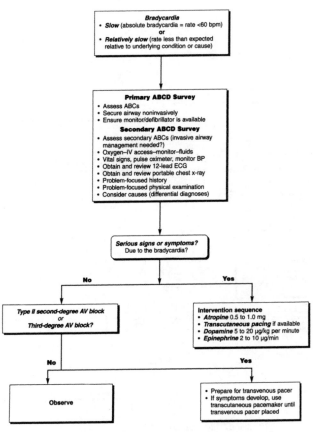

Figure 5. Bradycardia Algorithm.

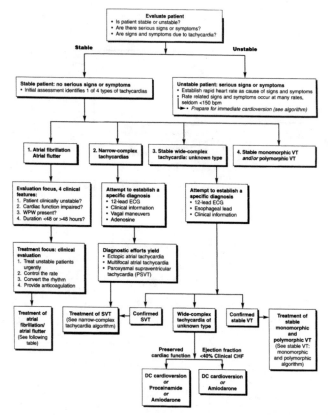

Figure 6. The Tachycardia Overview Algorithm.

Atrial fibrillation/ atrial flutter with • Normal heart • Impaired heart • WPW	1. Control Rate		2. Convert Rhythm	
	Heart Function Preserved	**Impaired Heart EF <40% or CHF**	**Duration <48 Hours**	**Duration >48 Hours or Unknown**
Normal cardiac function	Note: If AF >48 hours' duration, use agents to convert rhythm with extreme caution in patients not receiving adequate anticoagulation because of possible embolic complications. Use only 1 of the following agents (see note below): • Calcium channel blockers (Class I) • β-Blockers (Class I) • For additional drugs that are Class IIb recommendations, see Guidelines or ACLS text	(Does not apply)	**Consider** • DC cardioversion Use only 1 of the following agents (see note below): • Amiodarone (Class IIa) • Ibutilide (Class IIa) • Flecainide (Class IIa) • Propafenone (Class IIa) • Procainamide (Class IIa) • For additional drugs that are Class IIb recommendations, see Guidelines or ACLS text	• **NO DC cardioversion!** • Note: Conversion of AF to NSR with drugs or shock may cause embolization of atrial thrombi unless patient has adequate anticoagulation. • Use antiarrhythmic agents with extreme caution if AF >48 hours' duration (see note above). **or** *Delayed cardioversion* Anticoagulation × 3 weeks at proper levels • Cardioversion, then • Anticoagulation × 4 weeks more **or** *Early cardioversion* • Begin IV heparin at once • TEE to exclude atrial clot **then** • Cardioversion within 24 hours **then** • Anticoagulation × 4 more weeks
Impaired heart (EF <40% or CHF)	(Does not apply)	Note: If AF >48 hours' duration, use agents to convert rhythm with extreme caution in patients not receiving adequate anticoagulation because of possible embolic complications. Use only 1 of the following agents (see note below): • Digoxin (Class IIb) • Diltiazem (Class IIb) • Amiodarone (Class IIb)	**Consider** • DC cardioversion **or** • Amiodarone (Class IIb)	• Anticoagulation as described above, followed by • DC cardioversion
WPW	Note: If AF >48 hours' duration, use agents to convert rhythm with extreme caution in patients not receiving adequate anticoagulation because of possible embolic complications. • DC cardioversion **or** • Primary anti-arrhythmic agents Use only 1 of the following agents (see note below): • Amiodarone (Class IIb) • Flecainide (Class IIb) • Procainamide (Class IIb) • Propafenone (Class IIb) • Sotalol (Class IIb) --- *Class III (can be harmful)* • Adenosine • β-Blockers • Calcium blockers • Digoxin	Note: If AF >48 hours' duration, use agents to convert rhythm with extreme caution in patients not receiving adequate anticoagulation because of possible embolic complications. • DC cardioversion **or** • Amiodarone (Class IIb)	• DC cardioversion **or** • Primary anti-arrhythmic agents Use only 1 of the following agents (see note below**): • Amiodarone (Class IIb) • Flecainide (Class IIb) • Procainamide (Class IIb) • Propafenone (Class IIb) • Sotalol (Class IIb) --- *Class III (can be harmful)* • Adenosine • β-Blockers • Calcium blockers • Digoxin	• Anticoagulation as described above, followed by • DC cardioversion

WPW indicates Wolff-Parkinson-White syndrome; AF, atrial fibrillation; NSR, normal sinus rhythm; TEE, transesophageal echocardiogram; and EF, ejection fraction.

Note: Occasionally 2 of the named antiarrhythmic agents may be used, but use of these agents in combination may have proarrhythmic potential. The classes listed represent the Class of Recommendation rather than the Vaughn-Williams classification of antiarrhythmics.

Table 1. Control of Rate and Rhythm (Continued from Tachycardia Overview).

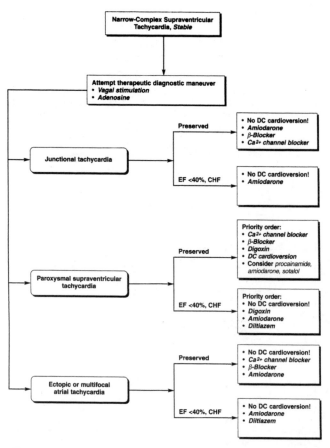

Figure 7. Narrow-Complex Supraventricular Tachycardia Overview.

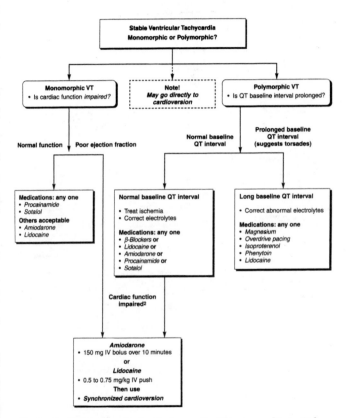

Figure 8. Stable Ventricular Tachycardia (Monomorphic or Polymorphic) Algorithm.

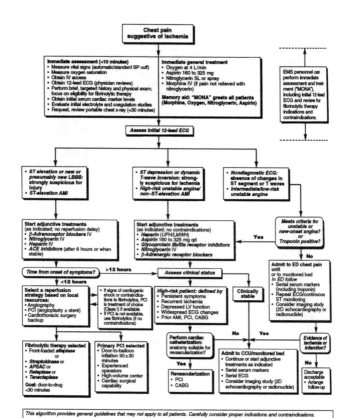

Figure 9. Acute Ischemic Chest Pain Protocol. Although local evaluation, diagnosis, and treatment may vary, core concepts involve the prompt treatment of ischemic-type chest pain with oxygen, nitrates, and morphine. The ECG is central to the initial triage of patients and allows identification of patients at high, intermediate, or low risk, who may then be further evaluated. Patients with ST-segment depression identifies a group of patients at high short-term risk for cardiac events, and aggressive antiplatelet therapy is indicated whether a medical or invasive strategy is chosen. Some patients at increased risk also have nondiagnostic or normal ECGs, and the use of cardiac markers, C-reactive protein, and functional studies allows additional risk stratification.

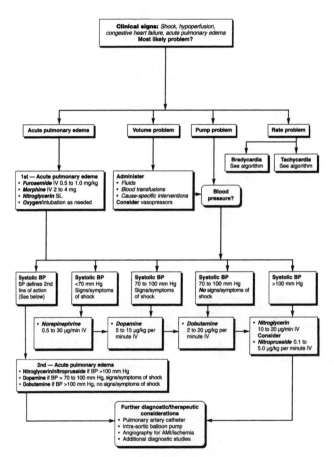

Figure 10. The Acute Pulmonary Edema, Hypotension, and Shock Algorithm.

B
APPENDIX

Effects of Specific Toxins on Various Organ Systems

VITAL SIGNS

Tachycardia: Ethanol, sympathomimetics, anticholinergics, theophylline, withdrawal states, salicylates, thyroid supplements, lithium, monoamine oxidase (MAO) inhibitors, digoxin, ergot alkaloids, TCAs, neuroleptics, mushrooms, nicotine

Bradycardia: Beta-blockers, calcium-channel blockers, barbiturates, cholinergics, sedatives and hypnotics, digitalis, opioids, CO, cyanide, cimetidine, clonidine, lead, organophosphates, quinine

Tachypnea: Anticholinergics, amphetamines, hydrocarbons, metabolic acidosis (**MUDPILES**), CO, salicylates, organophosphates, theophylline, withdrawal states, camphor, clonidine, cocaine, ethanol, methanol, ethylene glycol, hydrocarbons

Bradypnea: Alcohols, barbiturates, opioids, sedatives and hypnotics, clonidine, CO, cyanide (late exposure)

Hypertension: Anticholinergics, sympathomimetics, amphetamines, thyroid supplements, withdrawal states, barium, cadmium, CO, clonidine withdrawal, corticosteroids, ergot alkaloids, lead, mercury, MAO inhibitors, nicotine, theophylline

Hypotension: Antihypertensives, sedatives, opioids, TCAs, iron, CO, cyanide, digitalis, nitrites, nitrates, mushrooms, barbiturates, disulfiram (Antabuse), procainamide, insecticides, LSD

Hyperthermia: Anticholinergics, sympathomimetics,

phenothiazines, salicylates, TCAs, ethanol withdrawal, amphetamines, beta-blockers, atropine, iron, antihistamines, herbicides, metal fumes, thyroid supplements, theophylline, snake venom

Hypothermia: Barbiturates, opioids, sedatives, TCAs, alcohol, hypoglycemic agents, CO, cyanide, ethanol, clonidine, antipsychotics, hydrogen sulfide

NEUROLOGIC EXAMINATION

Miosis (pinpoint pupils): Use the mnemonic **POOPP:** **P** = PCP; **O** = opioids (except meperidine, diphenoxylate, dextromethorphan); **O** = organophosphates and cholinergics; **P** = phenothiazines; **P** = pontine hemorrhage. Also barbiturates (late) and nicotine

Mydriasis (dilated pupils): Use the mnemonic **SAW: S** = sympathomimetics; **A** = anticholinergics; **W** = withdrawal of substances of abuse. Also phenytoin, glutethimide, barbiturates, xanthines, cimetidine, and antihistamines

Seizures: Use the mnemonic **CAP: C** = carbon monoxide, camphor, cocaine, cyanide, chlorinated hydrocarbons; **A** = anticholinergics, aspirin, amphetamines/sympathomimetics, aminophylline, alcohols, ammonia, arsenic; **P** = PCP, phenothiazines, pesticides, phenytoin, propoxyphene, phenol. Also lead, lithium, carbamazepine, strychnine, antidepressants, and hypoglycemic agents

Nystagmus: Phenytoin, carbamazepine, barbiturates, glutethimide, salicylates, CO, alcohols, sedatives, PCP (often rotatory)

Toxic psychosis: Sympathomimetics, anticholinergics, hallucinogens, heavy metals, carbon disulfide

Violent behavior: PCP, cocaine, amphetamines, ethanol

THE SKIN

Cyanosis: Nitrates, nitrites, sulfonamides, aniline dyes

Dry, flushed skin: Anticholinergics, botulinum toxin

Profuse sweating: Cholinergics, anticholinesterases, sympathomimetics, salicylates, ethanol withdrawal, dinitrophenol

Bullae: Barbiturates, CO, ethchlorvynol, hexachlorbenzene, scombroid poisoning

Skin discoloration: *Blue:* oxalic acid; *bronze:* arsine; *brown:* bromides, iodine, nitrates, nitrites, phenytoin, local anesthetics; *gray-black:* chloramphenicol, silver; *orange:* nitric acid; *red:* antihistamines, anticholinergics, CO, cyanide, boric acid, rifampin, vancomycin, mercury; *yellow:* carotenoids, epoxy resins, rifampin

Needle tracks: Opioids, cocaine

Purpura: Anticoagulants, quinine, salicylates, snake and spider bites

Piloerection: Withdrawal states

DIAGNOSTIC ODORS

Acetone: Lacquer, alcohol, ketoacidosis, chloroform, isopropyl alcohol, phenol, salicylates

Bitter almonds: cyanide, silver polish

Stove gas: CO (odorless yet associated with stove gas)

Fruit-like: Amyl nitrite, chloral hydrate, ethanol

Rotten eggs: Hydrogen sulfide, disulfiram (Antabuse), mercaptens

Wintergreen: Methyl salicylate

Moth balls: Naphthalene, camphor

Shoe polish: Nitrobenzenes

Ammonia: Uremia

Garlic: Arsenic, organophosphates, selenium, malathion, parathion, thallium, dimethylsulfoxide

Index

An "f" following a page number indicates a figure;
a "t" indicates a table.